Fitnessworks!™

Jane Katz, EdD
The Bronx Community College
of the City University of New York

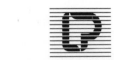

Leisure Press Publications
Champaign, Illinois

Cover Design: Conundrum Designs
Cover Photos By: Top: Focus West All Rights Reserved © 1987; Bottom
  Left: Tim Davis/Focus West All Rights Reserved © 1987; Bottom Right:
  David Lissy/Focus West All Rights Reserved © 1987
Back Cover Photo By: Fran Vogel
Photos in text: Page 1, by Jim Tiffany; page 23, by Fran Vogel; page 33,
  from University of California, Department of Women's Athletics;
  page 51, by David Lissy/Focus West, All Rights Reserved © 1987;
  page 63, by Tim Davis/Focus West, All Rights Reserved © 1987;
  page 81, by Ernie Noa
Printed By: Versa Press

ISBN: 0-88011-295-6

Copyright © 1988 by Jane Katz

FitnessWorks™, FootWorks™, WaterWorks™, CycleWorks™, and
NutritionWorks™ are trademarks of Jane Katz, EdD, for total health and
physical fitness products and services.

Library of Congress Cataloging-in-Publication Data

Katz, Jane.
  FitnessWorks!

  Bibliography: p.
  Includes index.
  1. Exercise. 2. Nutrition. 3. Physical fitness.
I. Title.
RA781.K3 1988   613.7   87-13576
ISBN 0-88011-295-6

Printed in the United States of America

10 9 8 7 6 5 4 3 2 1

Leisure Press
A division of Human Kinetics Publishers, Inc.
Box 5076, Champaign, IL 61820
1-800-DIAL-HKP
1-800-334-3665 (in Illinois)

Dedication

FitnessWorks! is dedicated to sports enthusiasts and new sports participants everywhere, both the young and the young at heart.

Editorial and production credits:

Developmental Editor: Sue Ingels Mauck
Copy Editor: Claire M. Mount
Assistant Editor: JoAnne Cline
Production Director: Ernie Noa
Projects Manager: Lezli Harris
Typesetter: Sandra Meier
Text Design: Keith Blomberg
Text Layout: Denise Mueller
Illustrations By: Keith Blomberg

Acknowledgments

I've been exercising all of my life as well as teaching and encouraging others to do the same. I hope this book will help others to join the fitness trend that has exploded throughout our country.

There have been many people who have supported and helped me in the development of *FitnessWorks*!

- My parents, Dorothea and Leon, who taught the joy of sport and who still have a joy of life.
- My other family members, Paul, Elaine, June, Joel, Stephen, Jason, and Justin, who have shared the joys of play with me at every age.
- Elaine Hochuli, MA, Therapeutic Recreation Specialist, whose input and enthusiasm have been forthcoming throughout the writing of the book.
- June Guzman, BS, Home Economics, Foods, and Nutrition, who contributed immensely to the NutritionWorks section.
- Arden Pilbro-Katz for her tasty CookWorks recipes.
- Marvin Cramer, MD, whose constructive comments were graciously submitted and who provided sports medicine expertise and the timely Foreword to this book.
- Anne Goldstein, who showed patience and adroitness in typing this manuscript, and Ricki Pollack and Howard Chislett, EdD, who added their editing expertise.

- Herbert Erlanger, MD, whose timely input and advice were invaluable.
- The staff at Human Kinetics Publishers, Inc., including Rainer Martens, PhD, publisher; Sue Wilmoth, PhD, director of Life Enhancement Publications; Claire M. Mount, copy editor; and especially my developmental editor Sue Ingels Mauck, for her selfless time, interest, support, and encouragement.
- Photographer Fran Vogel (back cover), and illustrator Keith Blomberg, who brought alive on paper the fun of exercising.
- All my friends and specialists for their specific sports input, particularly, Andrew Brett, Seth Brody, Millie Leinweber-Dawson, Luca del Borgo, Fran Hare, Stephen Jacoby, Steven Jonas, MD, Margaret Johnson, Morris Johnson, Ken Krueger, Jay Moskowitz, Willibald Nagler, MD, Elizabeth Nichol, Suzanne Rague, Ruben Riera, Betsy Tanner, Lila Wallis, MD, Leonard Waxman, and Helene Zimmerman.
- The Parks Department of the City of New York.
- And all the students whom I've had the pleasure to teach, and all the professional colleagues with whom I've enjoyed working and exercising.

Contents

Foreword

The past twenty years have seen a revolution in America's interest in physical fitness. Dr. Jane Katz has been one of the pioneers and leaders of this movement. "Dr. J" has been a member of the U.S. Masters All-American Swimming and Synchronized Swimming Teams since 1974 and continues to set world records. In her numerous books, magazine articles, and television appearances she has brought the same sort of enthusiasm, humor, and common sense to swimming that George Sheehan has brought to running.

My contact with Dr. Katz began when I read her book, *Swimming for Total Fitness* (1981), while I was making the transition from runner to triathlete. During the spring of 1986, I was asked to organize an exercise symposium at North Shore Hospital. I contacted experts from different backgrounds and I wanted a speaker on swimming. Every experienced swimmer I spoke to told me the same thing: "You've got to meet Jane Katz!" She agreed to come, and, as I expected, her lecture was a big success. Within a few minutes she had captivated the entire audience; everyone was practicing strokes as she demonstrated ways to improve them.

In *FitnessWorks!*, Dr. Katz expands her sports expertise to include a variety of aerobic activities. She provides valuable information for the neophyte as well as the returning exerciser.

With great support and encouragement, she guides the sports enthusiast into the exciting and rewarding activities of walking, running, cycling, and swimming.

The section on NutritionWorks follows up and enhances the FitnessWorks program by providing information for a healthy, well-balanced diet. In addition, an extensive question and answer section highlights common concerns. *FitnessWorks!* is a great starting point for anyone beginning a lifetime exercise program.

Marvin E. Cramer, MD
Cornell University, Department of Medicine
North Shore University Hospital, New York, NY

Preface

Physical fitness is one of the most frequent topics of conversation today. Everywhere you look, discussions of physical fitness and well-being fill the pages of magazines and books, and fitness professionals and nonprofessionals tout their particular programs for physical fitness. If you look out of your window, you can see neighbors jogging or walking down the street. And if you look a bit further, you'll probably find other people you know swimming laps at the local Y. Everyone is in hot pursuit of fitness. Although some view physical fitness as an imaginary fountain of youth, more realistic individuals recognize the connection between fitness and an improvement in their life-style, appearance, and well-being.

Two-thousand years ago, Hippocrates and Galen noted the relationship between physical fitness and well-being. Throughout the centuries, we have been told by physician and philosopher alike to care for our bodies and minds. As the ancient Romans used to say: *Mens sana in corpora sana* (''A healthy mind in a healthy body'').

Although there has been a gradual growth in interest in physical fitness over the years, it was in the late 1960s that Kenneth H. Cooper, MD popularized the positive connection between sustained exercise (aerobics) and cardiovascular health. Since that time the interest in fitness has continued to grow quite rapidly.

In 1972, the Olympic marathon was won by American Frank Shorter. In the same year the New York City Marathon attracted only a handful of runners and viewers. Through the seventies Americans got up from their easy chairs and began to rummage through their closets and attics in search of their old high school sneakers. By 1987, over twenty thousand runners of all ages and levels of ability participated in the New York City Marathon, making it one of the world's largest participatory sports events.

Joggers and runners are but one part of a larger movement. Other sports enthusiasts cycle, play tennis, lift weights, swim laps, golf, ski downhill or cross-country, and participate in aerobic dance classes. Yesterday's fitness fad has become an integral part of today's life-style.

Why is this so? One reason is that exercise has been shown to have positive effects on health for many people. In a recent study conducted at Stanford University, Dr. Ralph Paffenburger found that persons who participated in a moderate exercise program that used about 2,000 calories a week lessened their chances of developing life-threatening coronary problems by 30 percent.

Recent studies regarding exercise and aging suggest that the benefits of exercise are numerous and profound. For example, moderate exercise has been found to lower blood pressure and serum cholesterol, prevent or delay bone loss (osteoporosis), increase flexibility, decrease body fat, and help the body use oxygen more efficiently. It is probable that exercise may help to delay and/or prevent adult-onset diabetes and strokes.

Individuals who exercise tend to be leaner because exercise uses calories during and after activity. Besides the calories burned in the workout, exercise raises the metabolic rate so that the body continues to burn calories even while it is resting or sleeping. Exercise also helps reduce stress in the body as a whole; it helps to decrease depression, and gives a person a sense of well-being. These benefits improve the quality and enjoyment of life and, in some cases, prevent disease and injury.

Many studies indicate that low-intensity exercise programs improve cardiovascular fitness nearly as much as high-intensity programs. Therefore, the old saying, "no pain, no gain," no longer applies. So, don't worry if you're in the slow lane; you may be in the best lane.

You can make your exercise program more interesting and well-rounded by adding variety. Mix and match your activities so that you will be able to exercise different muscle groups. Try walking one day, then swimming, cycling, or running the next. All of these sports activities are included in the FitnessWorks program.

Make exercise and fitness an activity in which the entire family can participate in some form. Some of the happiest moments of my own life have been spent exercising with members of my family. A brisk walk together through your neighborhood, in the woods, or anywhere, can lead to all sorts of good things. The whole family can take bike rides together, with the smallest children riding in seats behind Mom and Dad. Also, your family can enjoy water sports and recreation at the local pool. The running boom has spawned "Fun Runs" in which all family members can participate because they are essentially noncompetitive— everyone is a winner. Involvement in these sports activities is often shared with others throughout life, thus resulting in the formation of meaningful bonds.

Although it seems that everyone is active, there are still millions of Americans who do not exercise on a regular basis. A recent report by the President's Council on Physical Fitness found that the fitness level of America's schoolchildren has not shown much improvement over the last decade. This study also showed that only 36 percent of school-age youngsters have daily physical education classes in their schools. School-age children, in particular, need to be indoctrinated early into the lifelong benefits of fitness. But it is also time for you to gear up and exercise. This book is for you!

Welcome to *FitnessWorks!*. In this book you will be introduced to a variety of aerobic exercises; most of them are low impact, easy to follow, and adaptable to your particular life-style. The most popular are walking/jogging, cycling, and swimming and water exercises. These are all highlighted. This approach will let you choose from among them so that you can improve your fitness and triple your fun.

Learn the fundamentals of exercising through TrainingWorks, which applies to all aerobic sports activities. Warm-up and cooldown stretches are included in this section. The OtherWorks section outlines exercises to do at home and at work. The FootWorks, WaterWorks, and CycleWorks sections provide the basics of each activity. The NutritionWorks section shows you what to eat and why, as well as how to attain a realistic, healthy eating plan.

The last section answers the questions that are commonly asked about training, sports activities, nutrition, and safety. An Appendix has been included to provide sources for further FitnessWorks information. So turn the page to the next and best chapter of your life, *FitnessWorks!*

Jane Katz, EdD
New York, NY

Introduction: Plunge Into FitnessWorks™

Exercise is play; it satisfies a need and creates a feeling of inner contentment. Exercise is pure pleasure that I want all of you to experience because it will help you look terrific, feel great, sleep better, and develop muscle tone and definition. You'll stand with a confident posture and feel exhilarated about yourself!

I started my love affair with sports when exercise was neither in fashion nor encouraged for young women. Fortunately I grew up in a family that fostered sports activities for everyone. Blossoming in a challenging urban setting, I took my first tricycle ride, running steps, and swim strokes in the beautiful parks of New York City. My professional career as a lecturer, author, champion swimmer, and professor of health and physical fitness stems from these early days.

Recent research has shown that low-impact aerobic exercise may be the best means for giving your cardiovascular system (heart and lungs) a workout. You can do this effectively by spend-ing approximately thirty minutes three times a week doing low-impact aerobics. So, get off the bench and cure your "spectator-itis." Give up the classic excuses: "It's too cold (or too hot)." "I have aches and pains." "I have no time." "The traffic was heavy." "I've lost my gym bag." I've heard them all in my 25 years of teaching at one of the largest universities in the country. Get off your duff, take the plunge, and become a minijock. You'll not only feel better, you'll look better. Instead of being a sports fan, be your own coach, player, and teammate. Create your own triathlon of sports activities. If you want to change your exer-cise, eating, or smoking habits and improve your overall health status, then this book is for you. Implement the following Foot-Works, WaterWorks, CycleWorks, and NutritionWorks to form your own FitnessWorks program.

See you sportside!

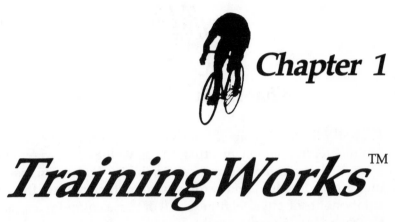

Chapter 1

Training Works™

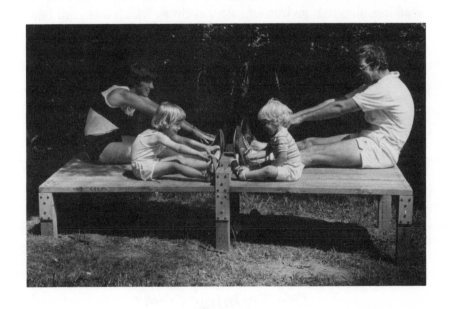

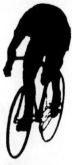

What Is Physical Fitness?

Physical fitness is the ability of the body to function at an optimum level in emergency situations as well as everyday living. Strength, muscular endurance, flexibility, body composition, motor coordination, and cardiovascular efficiency are the basic components of physical fitness. All of these components can be improved by doing the aerobic FitnessWorks activities, such as, walking, jogging, swimming, and cycling, which use your heart and lungs over a sustained period of time.

Strength is the capacity of a muscle to exert force against a resistance. *Endurance* allows the muscle to exert repeatedly a force or static contraction over a period of time. *Flexibility* is the range of motion of a specific joint and its corresponding muscle group. *Body composition* refers to the relative amounts of muscle, bone, and fat in a body. *Motor coordination* and *skill* are one's athletic ability, a combination of innate ability and practice.

Cardiovascular efficiency is the most important component of physical fitness. It is the capacity of your heart and lungs to function efficiently in order to bring oxygen to the tissues and remove waste products from the body. This component can be developed by applying the training effect (described below).

The Training Effect

The training effect began with the ancient Greek wrestler, Milo, who carried a calf around on his shoulders every day in order to become stronger. As the calf grew, Milo grew stronger and stronger. This illustrates the principle of progressive overload and how the body learns to adapt to increased demands of work.

To apply progressive overload in your FitnessWorks program, you exercise in a progressive fashion so that your body is better able to handle the stresses and strains of everyday living. Your blood vessels increase in number and your heart, like other muscles, becomes stronger. The skeletal muscle fibers, when exercised, become larger and stronger. In addition, they stretch and become more flexible!

Remember that the training effect takes time. You didn't get out of shape overnight, and it will take time for you to get back into condition. However, if you exercise three times a week for thirty minutes, in approximately eight to ten weeks, you will feel and see the training effect.

The Beat Goes On

Knowing your body's aerobic capacity means knowing your heart's vital statistics and what they mean. Your resting pulse rate registers your heart beat when you are not physically active (this is usually more accurately recorded in the morning before you get out of bed). Often as your physical fitness improves your resting pulse rate becomes lower; your heart processes the same amount of blood with less effort.

During aerobic activities your heart rate will increase. The harder you work the faster it gets. To find your aerobic activity heart rate you need to first find what is called your maximum heart rate (MHR). A simple formula to determine your MHR is 220 minus your age. Current research indicates that in order to benefit from aerobic activity, you need to exercise at 60-85 percent of your MHR and sustain it for approximately twenty minutes. You should begin at the lower end of this range when you begin an aerobic fitness program, and gradually increase toward the middle and higher end of your range.

This 60-85 percent range is called the target or training heart rate range (THR). THR is a concept that emerged from research in human fitness and is a personal guideline to help one safely achieve cardiovascular fitness. Exercising in this range will strengthen the heart, improve circulation, and lower blood pressure. To determine your THR range multiply your MHR (220 minus age) by .60. The middle part of the range, or approximately

75 percent of your MHR, is a reasonable goal to achieve during most workouts. The upper end of the range (your MHR multiplied by .85) should only be a goal for those in excellent physical condition.

Pulse Check

During your FitnessWorks, pause to take your pulse by gently placing your index finger on your wrist or on either side of your neck at the carotid artery (see Figure 1.1a and b). Count the beats for six seconds and multiply by ten (simply add a zero) to determine the number of beats per minute (e.g., if you count 14 beats, add a zero; your heart rate is 140).

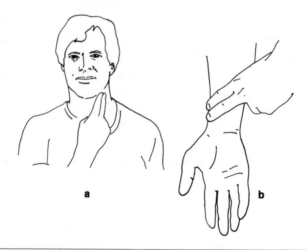

Figure 1.1. Location for checking heart rate: (a) carotid (neck) pulse, (b) radial (wrist) pulse.

Table 1.1 is an aerobic THR guide based on the equation to determine your target heart rate. It also provides figures for 75 percent of MHR. This midrange figure is a guide to aim for; your pulse may fall a few beats above or below this. In addition to checking your heart rate, remember to listen to your body, too. It may give you signals that you are working too hard: shortness of breath, muscle or joint pain, and other forms of discomfort.

Table 1.1   Aerobic Target Heart Rate (THR) Guide

Age	Maximum Beats per Minute (220 – Age)	THR: 60–85% of MHR in Beats per Minute	THR Goal 75% of MHR in Beats per Minute
20	200	120–170	150
25	195	117–166	146
30	190	114–162	142
35	185	111–157	139
40	180	108–153	135
45	175	105–149	131
50	170	102–145	127
55	165	99–140	124
60	160	96–136	120
65	155	93–132	116
70	150	90–128	112
75	145	87–123	109
80	140	84–119	105

Note. This 75% THR is a general guide for monitoring the main set of your workout. If you count a beat more or less within the six-second pulse count, you're still within your THR range (60-85%).

Your FitnessWorks Workout

Regardless of which activity you choose, you should follow the FitnessWorks workout. This includes a warm-up, a main set, and a cool-down.

The *warm-up* gets your body and mind in motion. Warm-up involves a gradual stretching of your muscles and a gradual increase in blood flow and heart rate (similar to warming up your car on a cold day). Your mind begins to concentrate on how your body is moving and feeling and psychs up for the workout. Your warm-up should take at least five minutes.

Your *main set* is the central part of the FitnessWorks workout. This means that you will be exercising aerobically for approximately twenty minutes. This is when you want to reach your target heart rate. Periodically check your pulse during the main set.

The *cool-down* helps your body to slow down, stretch out, and relax gradually. It brings your heart rate back to its normal resting rate. The cool-down should be at least five minutes.

Look at the heart rate pattern during a typical FitnessWorks workout in Figure 1.2. Use this as a guide for all workouts.

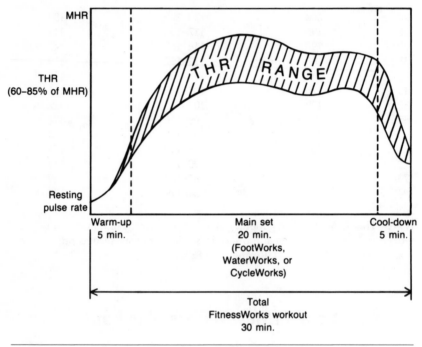

Figure 1.2. Heart rate pattern during a typical FitnessWorks workout.

TrainingWorks Concepts: The F.I.T. Principle

To achieve an aerobic training effect, you need to overload your body gradually by increasing the frequency, intensity, and time of your workout. I call this the F.I.T. principle. Research has shown that to benefit from your program you should work out at least three times a week on alternate days of the week for approximately thirty minutes. However, there are several ways to enhance and vary your workout.

Frequency: Increase the number of workouts per week (to four or more). For variety, alternate your activities (one day each of WaterWorks, FootWorks, and CycleWorks).

Intensity: Change your main set with variations of training techniques and equipment (changing bicycle gears, using swim fins, and increasing distance). Challenge yourself with a different environment (e.g., hills, open water, different terrain).

Time: Increase your workout by combining two activities (cycle or walk to the pool). Shorten the length and/or decrease the number of your rest periods in your main set. Gradually increase the length of your main set.

TrainingWorks Variations

Variety is beneficial for many aspects of life, and it also applies to your FitnessWorks program. Here are three ways to train, so you can triple your fitness and your fun!

Continuous, Consistent Movement

Exercise at approximately the same rate or speed without stopping during a twenty-minute aerobic main set. Pacing is the key: You need to begin and hold a comfortable speed of motion. For example, cycle for twenty minutes at a consistent pace.

Fartlek Training

Fartlek is a Swedish word meaning *speed play*. *Fartlek* training has been widely used among runners as a training technique but can be applied to all FitnessWorks activities. This technique basically employs alternating speeds during a workout session (e.g., variations of slow, medium, and fast). For this method your THR should reach approximately 75 percent of its maximum rate during the fast phase. For example, walk slowly for one minute, walk briskly for one minute, and then jog for one minute, repeat.

Interval Training

This method of training is the most efficient for improving aerobic fitness. For this method, periods of intense training are interspersed with brief rest periods. For example, swim twenty-five yards every minute. Repeat this cycle four times (e.g., if you complete twenty-five yards in forty seconds, you will rest twenty seconds before you start the next twenty-five-yard swim). So, the faster you swim, the longer the rest period will be.

These TrainingWorks variations can be mixed and matched in many ways, and they can be applied to the F.I.T. principle. Using a variety of training techniques can help maintain your motivation and enthusiasm for FitnessWorks.

Motivation Is the Key for Fitness Success

If you are a weekend athlete or if you have devised a number of excuses for avoiding exercise, then you need a realistic outlook when it comes to exercise. When you begin a fitness program, you need to set attainable goals and design a program that is flexible enough to fit into your schedule. Rather than saying, "If I only had time," you need to make the time for exercise in the course of your day. If you have a difficult time finding one-half hour per day three times per week, reevaluate the time you spend on the telephone or watching television. Whether you prefer to exercise in the morning, at lunchtime, or at the end of the day, build your exercise program around the time of day that suits you best.

Here are more tips for getting motivated to exercise.

- Exercise with a friend or family member.
- Join a regular fitness workout class, group, or facility. When you've paid your membership dues, you often feel obligated to use the facility.
- Gear up with new fitness toys to enhance your program and provide increased motivation.
- Learn more about your FitnessWorks exercises through clubs, organizations, clinics, and publications. (See Source-Works for specifics.)
- Watch elite and professional athletes—live or on TV. You can learn a great deal from their techniques, and you can appreciate their efforts more.
- Log your aerobic progress to have a record of what you've done and how much you have improved.

- Remember, including FitnessWorks in your daily life will help you feel better and look better.

Let's get started with FitnessWorks warm-ups. StretchWorks has been designed to accompany any of the FitnessWorks activities. Be sure to pay attention to the safety reminders. Go over each one prior to the start of your FitnessWorks program.

FitnessWorks Safety Reminders

1. Remember this book is not a substitute for consulting your physician. Before beginning this FitnessWorks program (or any other aerobic program), you should have a medical checkup if you
   - don't exercise regularly or are a weekend athlete,
   - are over the age of thirty-five,
   - have recently recovered from an injury or surgery, or
   - have a health problem.
2. Always listen to your body and never push yourself to extreme discomfort.
3. Remember to warm up before your main set and to cool down afterwards.
4. Refrain from your FitnessWorks when you're injured, sick, or very tired.
5. Monitor your pulse during your main set.
6. Be sure you're comfortable at your present level before you proceed to the next step of any FitnessWorks activity.

StretchWorks

These StretchWorks exercises (Figures 1.3 through 1.12) are designed for you to do as the warm-up and cool-down parts of your workout. Allow approximately five minutes at the beginning and at the end of your workout for StretchWorks. Perform each exercise for approximately fifteen to thirty seconds. Move into each position with continuous motion. Feel your muscles ease into the stretch. You should not experience any excessive discomfort or pain.

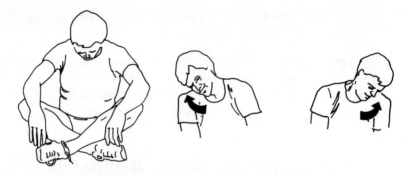

Figure 1.3. *Head semicircles.* Nod head forward, chin to chest, then rotate sideward, to the left, back to the chest, and then to the right shoulder. Do two semicircles in each direction. This helps to stretch neck muscles.

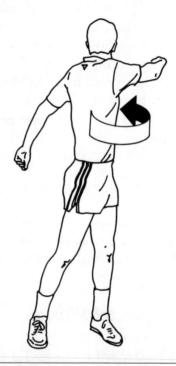

Figure 1.4. *Body twist.* Stretch your arms straight overhead. Clasp your hands and slowly twist your body to the right, allowing left knee to bend slightly. Twist to the left, allowing right knee to bend slightly. Continue twisting with hands on hips, alternating right to left. Then twist with arms stretched out sidewards at shoulder height. Twist slowly and continuously doing each of the three variations ten times each. This stretches the muscles of the shoulders and torso.

Whenever you stretch or perform other similar exercises, remember to feel the stretch in your muscles, not ligaments or joints, avoid locking or overbending your joints, avoid bouncing or arching your lower back or neck, and swing arms and legs slowly and continuously.

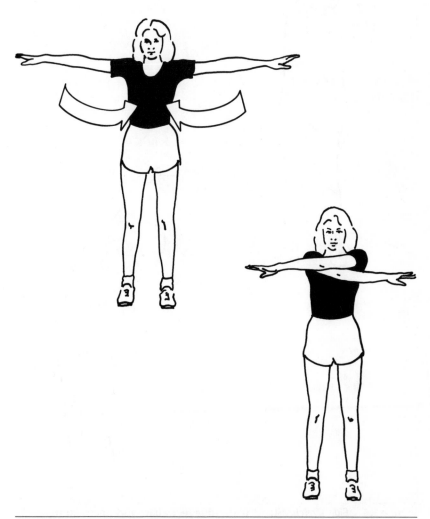

Figure 1.5. *Arm stretch.* Stretch your arms out sideward at shoulder height. With elbows locked (straight), bring arms forward crossing them in front of your body. Then bring arms together behind you, crossing them if possible. Stretch arms forward to backward to forward continuously for sixteen cycles. This stretches the back, arms, and chest muscles.

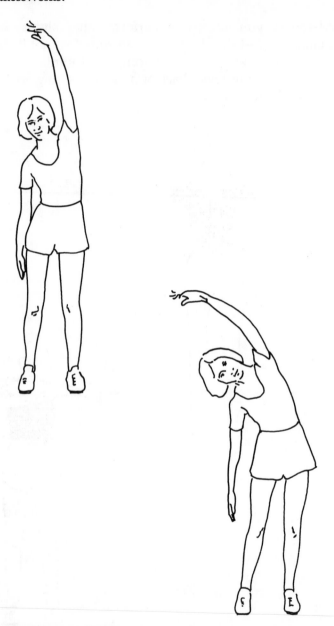

Figure 1.6. *Side stretch.* Stand with your feet apart and knees straight. Start with both hands along the sides of your thighs, then stretch your right arm straight overhead. Slide your left hand slowly down your leg. Your body will bend to the left. Hold the bend for at least fifteen seconds and then stretch to the right. This stretches the muscles of the upper body.

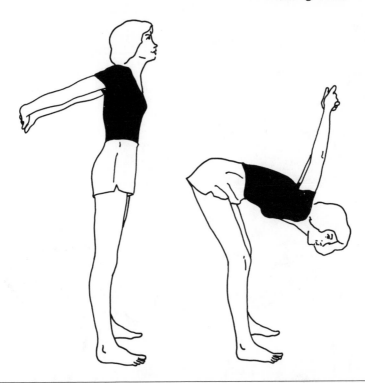

Figure 1.7. *Arm and hamstring stretch.* Stand straight with your feet apart. Clasp your hands behind your back. Inhale, lifting your arms up. Exhale and lower arms. Then bend torso forward from hip, keeping knees slightly bent. Stretch arms up. Hold back straight, abdomen pulled in. Hold for fifteen seconds. Return upright. Repeat. This stretches the arms and the hamstring muscles (back of thighs).

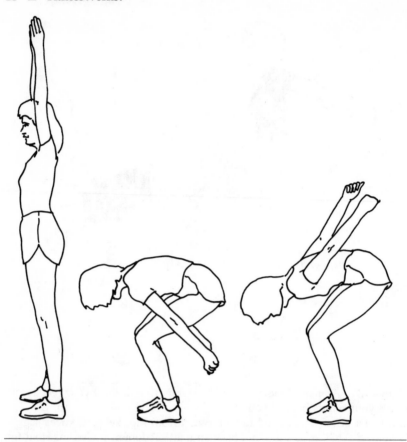

Figure 1.8. *Body swing*. Stand and stretch your arms overhead. Drop arms forward bending body downward, head between bent knees. Then bring torso and arms back up to standing position. Repeat ten times. This stretches the lower back muscles.

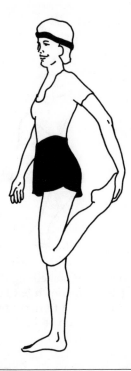

Figure 1.9. *Thigh stretch.* Stand holding onto something that is stationary with right hand. Bend left foot up to buttock. Reach left hand behind you, grasping left ankle and hold fifteen seconds. Repeat on right side. You will feel this stretch in the thigh or quadriceps muscles. When performing this stretch, you should not feel pressure or pain in the bent knee.

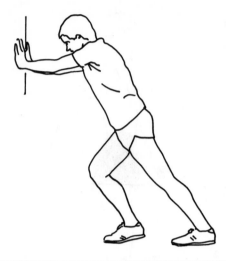

Figure 1.10. *Lower leg stretch.* Hold something that is stationary. Point your right foot forward, knee bent; stretch left leg straight back, heel pressed against floor. Hold for fifteen to thirty seconds. Repeat on other leg. This stretches the Achilles tendon and calf muscle.

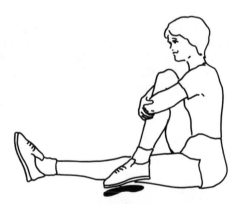

Figure 1.11. *Buttock stretch.* Sit on floor with your legs together and your knees straight. Cross right foot over left leg, placing right foot on the ground, as close to your hip as possible. Wrap arms around right knee pulling it toward your chest. Hold for fifteen to thirty seconds. Repeat on other leg. This stretches the gluteus muscle group.

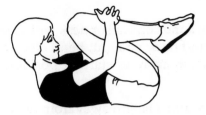

Figure 1.12. *Back stretch.* Lie on your back and bring both knees to your chest. Bring chin toward chest. Grasp your shins and pull the knees to your face. Hold for fifteen to thirty seconds. This stretches the back and neck muscles.

Staying Fit in Place

In your daily life there are times when traveling, home responsibilities, and work limit your time, space, and energy to exercise. Here are some exercises you can do on the job, at home, or when traveling, to help ease your stress and re-energize your mind and body.

JobWorks

If your work routine is sedentary, exercising during your work day, for as little as ten minutes a day, can do wonders for your mind and spirit. When you sit at a desk or computer terminal all day you can become stiff and somewhat tense, as well as less productive. Unfortunately, some of you may not be able to get away for a jog or a trip to a health club during the work day. I suggest taking a brief walk and/or doing the following exercises at your work station.

Posture Check and Breathing
Sit tall with your back against the chair. Grasp hands under chair, pulling upward as you inhale. Exhale and relax.

Shoulder Shrug
Shrug shoulders up and down. Then circle shoulders forward and backward.

Push-Away
Stand and place hands on wall or desk with arms extended. With heels on floor and body straight, bend elbows to bring chest to wall or desk. Push away to starting position.

Side Stretch
Stand sideways, arm's length away from desk, placing extended right hand on desk edge. Keep feet together. Bend right elbow, lean, and touch right hip to desk. Repeat five times and change sides.

Arm Circles
Stand with arms extended sideways at shoulder height, palms up. Circle each arm backward separately, making small circles. Repeat, circling forward.

Knee Tuck for Buttocks
Stand and hold chair for balance. Bend outside knee; lift and swing other leg forward and backward in a pumping motion. If your clothing restricts such movement try a "sitting bun squeeze." While you are sitting, press your buttocks together and hold for fifteen seconds. Relax, repeat.

Sit 'n Kick
Sitting in a chair with back straight; extend legs forward, parallel to floor. Alternately lift and lower legs up and down in a flutter-kick motion. Vary with a scissors action. Separate legs in a "V" position and then cross right over left. Repeat by crossing left leg over right.

OtherWorks

Use the following homework exercises to help complement your FitnessWorks program.

Jump Rope
This exercise is strenuous and most appropriate for the experienced exerciser. Use anything from a clothesline to a sophisticated leather jump rope with handles containing ball bearings and a counter. Jumping rope is a great endurance builder and cardiovascular strengthener.

Rebounders

Rebounders, or mini-trampolines are used to help absorb the impact characteristic of stationary jogging, jumping rope, and aerobic dance exercise. As with other aerobic activities, start at a comfortable pace and progressively increase your workout.

Calisthenics

A good routine of active calisthenics can be effective in promoting and maintaining aerobic fitness. Exercise to your favorite music. Remember to use the stretches in your warm-up as well as in your cool-down. Try following along with a TV exercise program.

Free Weights

These can be used to strengthen muscles. Use them in combination with your FitnessWorks.

Rowing Machines

Rowing machines exercise the shoulders, back, and legs and can provide all-around aerobic exercise. Gradually adjust the resistance of the oar pull so that you can progress in your workout.

Stationary Bike

See chapter 3, CycleWorks for more information.

Table 1.2 Sample FitnessWorks Week

Day	Morning	Noon	Afternoon	Evening
Monday	Jobworks*			
Tuesday		Walk/Jog		
Wednesday	Jobworks*			
Thursday				Cycle
Friday	Jobworks*			
Saturday			Swim	
Sunday		Swim		

*Optional

Mix and Match Your FitnessWorks

Table 1.2 shows a sample FitnessWorks week to help develop your total FitnessWorks program. There are cross-training effects whenever you are involved in more than one activity and you have the added benefit of variety in your FitnessWorks to help you stay motivated. Remember that you can exercise at different times of the day. Choose the FitnessWorks activities according to your schedule.

FitnessWorks Training Log

A training log like the one in Table 1.3 will help you chart your workout pattern. It's a great motivator to see your progress and improvement, particularly if you are just starting your Fitness-Works program. (Turn to Appendix B for a blank copy of the Training Log.)

Table 1.3 FitnessWorks Training Log

Date	Resting Pulse	FitnessWorks Activity	Warm-Up Pulse	Main Set Pulse	Cool-Down Pulse	Total Time/ Distance	Comments			
9/15 6pm	60	Cycling	90	146	85	36 minutes 6 miles	Felt Great			
9/17 6:30pm	62	Jogging	95	150	80	22 minutes 2.5 miles	Tired at First			
9/19 6pm	60	Swimming	90	145	85	6 laps 20 minutes	Felt Relaxed			

Chapter 2

FootWorks™

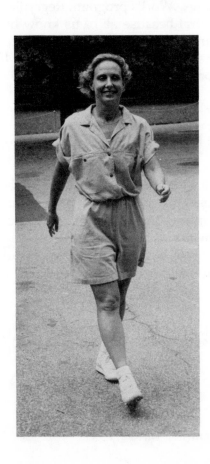

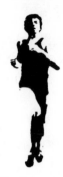

Go Take a Walk

In September of 1985, as a special consultant to the President's Council on Physical Fitness and Sports, I had the pleasure of presenting the Council's award to Rob Sweetgall, who successfully completed a fifty-state walk across America to promote the great benefits of walking. Walking is a very logical and safe way to begin your FitnessWorks program. Regardless of your fitness level, it is a natural because all of us know how to do it; and it can be done anywhere and at virtually any time. It is low impact, easy on the body, and good for the soul. If you have been inactive for a long time, then walking should be your starting point.

Gear Up for Walking

A wristwatch is useful for timing your walks and taking your pulse. Use a digital watch or one with a sweep second hand. Your only important gear is a good pair of shoes. A number of excellent shoes are now on the market. A pair of athletic shoes (e.g., jogging shoes or sneakers) is adequate. If you decide to become a more serious walker, then you should check out the wide variety of specially designed shoes for walking (see Figure 2.1).

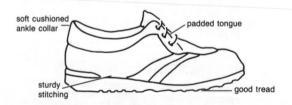

Figure 2.1. Anatomy of a walking shoe.

To go along with your shoes, you will need socks to give you added foot comfort and help absorb foot perspiration. If you're purchasing socks, stick to natural fibers such as cotton for warm weather and wool for cooler weather.

One of the great things about walking is that you can wear your everyday casual clothes—you don't need to purchase anything else. However, there are different types of clothing that have been designed for joggers that are equally useful for a walker. For example, some of the Gore-Tex jogging suits are great in cold and foul weather. Ultimately, gearing up for walking means getting a good pair of shoes; other than that, let common sense and the elements help determine what you will wear when you walk.

Walking is a safe place to begin your FootWorks program; it is hard to overdo, it's easy to stick with, and you can alternate it with jogging or other sports activities in your FitnessWorks.

Walking Basics—One Step at a Time

Stand with your feet hip-distance apart. Your head should be erect and slightly forward, back straight, and hands hanging loosely at your sides with fingers relaxed. Your knees should be slightly bent. Check your posture in a mirror.

Step forward with your heel touching first, toes pointed upward at a thirty to forty-five-degree angle. Remember to keep your hips in line with your torso. Swing your arms in an alternate pattern as you walk (as your right leg steps forward, your left arm will naturally swing forward too). Walk as naturally as possible. Inhale and exhale fully through both your nose and mouth. Remember to breathe rhythmically and comfortably as you walk. Finally, to get maximum aerobic benefits from walking, you need to maintain a comfortable but brisk striding pace of 3 to 5 miles per hour. This pace falls between 20 and 12 minutes per mile.

You can develop other walking interests such as hiking and backpacking. Enjoy the great outdoors on foot!

Go for a Jog

Perhaps no other form of physical exercise has so captured the American heart as jogging. The phenomenal number of people who take part in marathons reflects the tremendous interest millions of people have in jogging for fitness. Jogging is popular because it is a great exercise, which uses the large muscle groups of your legs and lower back. It can also burn more calories than most exercises in a shorter period of time.

Gear Up for Jogging

The most important equipment you will need is shoes. A good pair of running shoes is important; your feet are going to carry you down those roads and up those hills, and good shoes will make the trip a lot easier. Dismiss the idea of running in anything other than jogging shoes. Basketball sneakers, tennis shoes, boat shoes, and walking shoes are specific for their activity, but they are not good for jogging or running.

When you buy your jogging shoes, go in the late afternoon when your feet have had a chance to swell. Take a pair of athletic socks. Ask the salesperson to measure your foot while you are standing. Measure the length from heel to longest toe; the width is measured at the widest part of the ball of the foot.

Your shoes should have a good tread design for traction in wet or snowy weather. The shoe sole (outer and midsole) should be thick enough to provide cushioning and absorb shock, but not so thick as to be inflexible. To check this your shoe should bend easily in your hands. A rigid heel counter is also an important characteristic of a good shoe. The insole, where your foot rests, should be soft and yielding with a good arch support. A good test for roominess is to wiggle your toes in the shoes. There should be enough give so that all your toes are free to move. The shoe should also fit firmly around your heel with no sliding. Ask the shoe salesperson in the sporting goods store for advice on the proper running shoe for your needs and budget (see Figure 2.2).

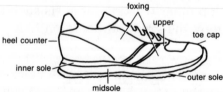

Figure 2.2. Anatomy of a running shoe.

You can expect to pay from about $30 to $75 or more for a pair of jogging shoes. Ultimately, you are the best judge of the shoe you buy. Try on several different pairs and move around to get the feel of them.

Sock It to You
Always wear socks to absorb foot perspiration. Choose your socks according to the weather. In warm weather, cotton socks are best. In cold weather, wool, or a combination of wool and silk, is a good choice. Wool and silk both have the ability to keep their insulating properties when damp.

Bottoms Up
Wear shorts or pants that allow freedom of movement. It's a good idea for them to have a pocket for your keys and some change for the telephone if necessary. There are also wrist and shoe holders available for these small items.

Top It Off
In warm weather, a nylon tank top or light cotton T-shirt is the most comfortable for jogging. In colder weather, wear several layers of light clothing. Check out the innumerable styles and types of cold-weather gear, from polypropylene underwear to Gore-Tex outerwear.

Head and Hand Gear
In warm weather, headbands or sun visors help to keep perspiration from running into your eyes. Cold weather calls for a knitted cap to avoid loss of body heat through your head.

Use a pair of gloves or mittens in colder weather. Wear a wristwatch, preferably with a sweep second hand so that you don't shortchange your FootWorks by not verifying your pulse rate.

Jogging How-To's

Position
Run with body erect and relaxed, keeping your head up. Lean your body slightly forward. Run with your elbows bent at ninety degrees, arms swinging easily, with hands relaxed. Each foot should strike the ground at the heel and roll forward (see Figure 2.3). Avoid overstriding and running on your toes.

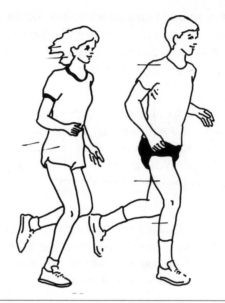

Figure 2.3. Proper running form.

Talk Test

Breathe naturally and rhythmically. To be certain you're comfortable, try the *talk test*. If you can carry on a conversation while you're jogging, then you are jogging at the correct pace; if you cannot carry on a conversation, slow down, you're moving too fast.

Safety Tips for FootWorks

1. Look out for hazards: dogs, cars, bikers, skaters, and other exercisers.
2. Avoid jogging on a full stomach.
3. Go to the bathroom before you begin.
4. Avoid brisk walking or jogging in the heat of the day.
5. Dress appropriately for cold weather.
6. Train—don't strain. Heed all aches and pains that don't go away.
7. Always remember to stretch with your warm-up and cool-down exercises.

8. Monitor your pulse rate to be sure you're in your THR range.
9. If you walk or jog before sunrise or after dark, use a jogging vest made from reflective material, or attach a piece of reflective tape to your hat, gloves, and the backs of your shoes so that you will be visible to drivers.
10. Face traffic when jogging on the roadside.
11. It is very important to listen to your body and choose the sport skills you like. You may wish to continue with your walking program and/or combine it with jogging.
12. Try to jog on giving surfaces, such as grass or special running tracks, to lessen strain on your joints.
13. To increase your FootWorks progressively, increase your walking and/or jogging distance by no more than 10 percent of your previous distance.
14. Use the following 10-Step Progressive FootWorks Program and stay on a step until you're ready to go on to the next one comfortably.

FootWorks Suggestions

1. Walk to work, if possible.
2. Explore your neighborhood/community.
3. Do errands during your walk.
4. Try exercising at different times of the day: before work, during lunch hour, after work.
5. Try to recruit a co-worker, friend, or family member to join you.
6. Don't let rain deter you from going out to walk or run. Dress accordingly.
7. Any time you see a staircase, walk up or down instead of using the elevator or escalator.
8. Try a *parcourse* (pronounced par-coors). A *parcourse* is any designated stretch of territory along which you alternately jog and then stop to do other stationary exercises. The activities combine cardiovascular exercise such as jogging with calisthenics. This helps to break up your exercise routine so it is more interesting and varied. You can develop

your own *parcourse*. Be creative at a playground using monkey bars, fences, benches, or poles.

9. Try skipping rope.
10. Do your FootWorks program in a park, historic area, or golf course (during off hours).
11. Vary the terrain. Try to run on grass, dirt, or on a track. These surfaces are much softer than cement or asphalt.
12. Walk or jog on a treadmill, if available. Depending on the model, you can vary your speed and elevation.
13. Bounce on a rebounder. It is a small trampoline with tighter springs. It allows you to jump up and down while the springs absorb the shock of your body's weight when you land.

10
STEP
Progressive FootWorks Program

STEP 1

Walk for twenty minutes. Gradually increase the distance you cover in a twenty-minute session.

STEP 2

Walk briskly for twenty minutes. Try including some short distances of jogging (approximately one block). Jog on the downhill slopes of your course or on the home stretch.

STEP 3

Jog one minute, walk three minutes; repeat four more times.

STEP 4

Jog three minutes, walk two minutes; repeat three more times.

STEP 5

Walk five minutes, jog five minutes, walk five minutes, jog five minutes.

STEP 6

Jog ten minutes, walk five minutes, jog five minutes.

STEP 7

Run two miles. Use a track or particular measured destination. Plan four *break stations* or predetermined landmarks where you can rest briefly, but keep walking. Don't stop completely. Try to use a half-mile distance as a guide. Record your total running time.

STEP 8

Jog six minutes, walk one minute; repeat two more times.

STEP 9

Jog for twenty minutes. Plan two break stations at which to walk for one minute each.

STEP 10

Jog for twenty minutes. Maintain a steady pace without any breaks.

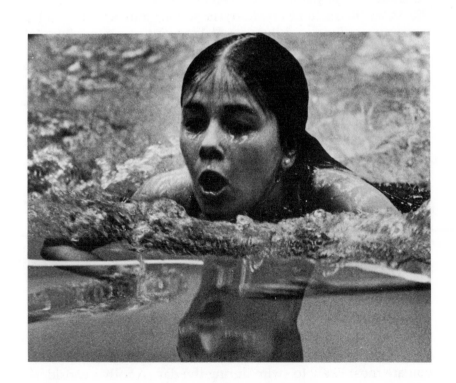

Chapter 3

WaterWorks™

Take the Plunge!

WaterWorks is for everyone! Swimming is the nation's number one recreational activity. Water is the perfect medium for exercising, toning up, relaxing, and simply having fun. In addition, water's buoyancy reduces your apparent body weight to 10 percent of your actual weight. For example, if you weigh 150 pounds on land, your apparent body weight will be only 15 pounds in the water! Because of this buoyancy, your movements will be graceful and fluid and little stress is placed on your joints. In general, exercising in the water improves your flexibility, strength, and aerobic conditioning.

Getting Started

The basic thing you need is a pool, lake, or other body of water. If you haven't found a source, try the following:

- YMCA, YWCA and YMHA, YWHA
- Schools and universities
- Private swim and health clubs
- Municipal, county, park and recreation departments
- A friend's backyard pool
- Pool listings in the yellow pages

The choice of an aquatic facility requires, first of all, a consideration of its schedule: when it is open during the week. This must be compatible with your own schedule, taking into account when you are most likely to swim during the day. Another consideration is location: Ideally, the facility should be close to your job and/or your home. If cost is a factor, consider a public or community pool, which is likely to be inexpensive or free. The size and depth of the water is also important. If you want to focus on water exercises, a small shallow pool is ideal. If you want to swim laps, look for a standard twenty-five-yard pool. Check the cleanliness of the facility. Also check to see if the facility provides the following: class schedules, piped-in music, lockers, proper atmosphere, exercise room, sauna, whirlpool, lap-swimming lanes, and other amenities.

Gear Up

In most cases, a swimsuit is a must. The latest in swimwear is a suit made of a combination of materials, usually nylon and lycra which is quick drying, durable, and comfortable. Prices for swimsuits can range from $15-$50 for women and $7-$20 for men. Although not necessary, the following equipment and swim toys are suggested to make your WaterWorks more enjoyable and effective:

- goggles (especially for lap swimmers) to help protect your eyes and help you to see clearly
- a pace clock; if unavailable, use a waterproof watch
- a lycra or latex swim cap (or sweat band) to keep your hair relatively dry and out of your face
- a kickboard (flotation device) to support your upper body so you can isolate your leg motion (Figure 3.1)

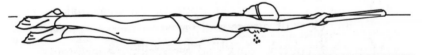

Figure 3.1. Kickboards and swim fins can add variety to your Water-Works workout.

- a pull-buoy (small styrofoam float) to support your legs so you can isolate your arm motion (Figure 3.2)
- fins to increase ankle flexibility and leg strength (Figure 3.1)
- hand paddles, which are resistance devices to strengthen your arms and upper body (Figure 3.2)

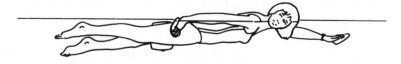

Figure 3.2. Pull-buoys and hand paddles can also aid your workout.

- water buoyancy support (e.g., vests, cushions, and other flotation devices) for aqua jogging

Breathing Is Basic

Try some homework for your WaterWorks. Practice rhythmic breathing in several inches of tap water in the privacy of your own home (e.g., sink, tub, large bowl). See Step 2 of the 10-Step Progressive WaterWorks Program for instructions for rhythmic breathing.

Safety Tips and Suggestions for WaterWorks

Before taking the plunge, you should observe the following safety tips:

1. Never swim alone.
2. Swim in an area that is appropriate to your ability.
3. Be aware of potential hazards in open water such as currents, rocks, pollution, and unmarked depths.
4. Do water exercises in an appropriate area, making sure to stay clear of divers and lap swimmers.
5. Check the water's depth before entering.
6. Swim in the lane that is most appropriate for you (when lanes are designated "slow," "medium," and "fast").
7. Always stay to the right of the lane when swimming laps (make your turns counter-clockwise).
8. When resting at the pool edge, keep to one side of the lane to allow other swimmers to turn easily.
9. Pass slower swimmers on the left; try to pass at the turns.
10. Check your pulse periodically to be sure your heart rate is in the target range. Your THR will be approximately 10% lower when exercising in the water.

10
STEP
Progressive WaterWorks Program

The following WaterWorks program is a 10-step progression. Depending on your level of fitness and your water skills, start and stay with the appropriate step until you feel comfortable enough to progress to the next step. Remember to warm up for five minutes before you start and to cool down for another five minutes after you finish your WaterWorks. A locker room or deck area is fine to do your StretchWorks.

Each of the following steps consists of several skills to perform in sequence. Remember, your main set should last at least twenty minutes; rest as needed between activities. Before you begin your WaterWorks activity, explore the pool or swimming area: Be aware of pool depths, ladder locations, and equipment availability.

Although the following steps focus on the crawl stroke, any of the basic swimming strokes may be used (breaststroke, back stroke, etc.). Choose the one you like best.

Lap length designations:
  20-yard pool: five lengths = 100 yards
  25-yard pool: four lengths = 100 yards
  50-meter pool: two lengths = 100 meters

STEP 1

Static arm and leg stretch (five minutes): Hold onto the pool wall with your left hand and place your left foot on the edge (see Figure 3.3). Stretch your right arm over your head toward the extended foot and hold for twenty seconds. Alternate feet.

Bobbing with breathing (five minutes): First practice breathing with just your chin on the water's surface. Inhale and exhale through your nose and mouth. Next, take a breath and place lips in the water and exhale, creating bubbles.

When you can perform this easily, try combining bobbing and breathing. Stand in chest-deep water and take a breath of air.

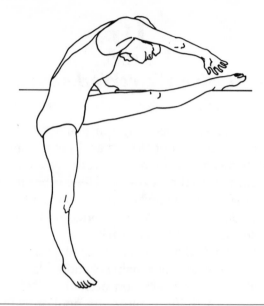

Figure 3.3. Static arm and leg stretch.

Bob under the surface submerging your body and head. Exhale the breath of air completely through your nose and mouth while submerged (see Figure 3.4). In order to exhale completely, try giving a big sigh. When exhaling correctly you should not become out of breath. Surface after exhaling. Try bobbing and breathing continuously, working up to ten times.

Water walk (five minutes): Walk in chest-deep water, using wall, kickboard, or rope for added balance if needed.

Aqua jog (five minutes): Stand in chest-deep water. Maintain your balance by placing palms down with arms flexed at the elbow at ninety degrees. Jog the width of the pool.

STEP **2**

Rhythmic breathing (five minutes): This technique will be used for the crawl stroke. Practice by standing in chest- to waist-deep water, holding onto the pool edge with both hands for support. Place one ear on the water's surface (see Figure 3.5). Inhale, making sure that your lips are out of the water. Then turn your head, placing your face in the water at hairline level, and exhale fully,

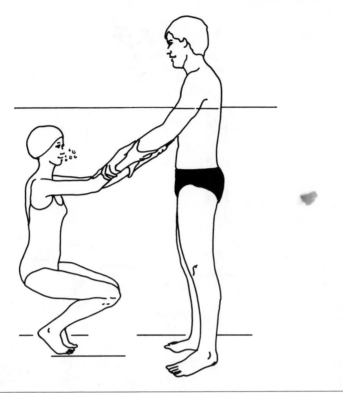

Figure 3.4. Bobbing with breathing.

forming bubbles. Turn your head again to the same side so your lips are out of the water and inhale. Exhale again with face in water. Practice until this rhythmic breathing feels comfortable.

Crawl armstroke while standing and walking (five minutes): The crawl armstroke is an alternating motion of the arms. One arm pulls straight underwater giving propulsion, while the other is lifted out of the water keeping the elbow bent above the water's surface and extending the hand forward in order to begin the next stroke. As the right arm pulls through the water for propulsion, the left arm recovers to start the next pull.

Practice this armstroke while standing and then while walking in chest-deep water.

Prone float and recovery to a stand (five minutes): This skill is used to stand up safely from a (front) floating position. Press your hands from an overhead, extended position downward toward

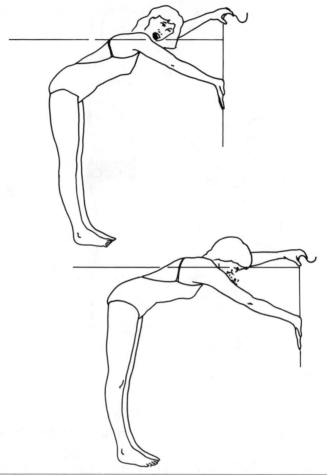

Figure 3.5. Rhythmic breathing.

your feet and the bottom of the pool while you lift your head and bend your knees and waist (see Figure 3.6a and b). When first performing this exercise, hold onto the wall, a partner's hands, or a kickboard for support.

Swim and/or water walk for a total of one minute, resting as needed.

STEP **3**

Flutter kick with rhythmic breathing (five minutes): Practice rhythmic breathing while grasping one edge of a kickboard or the pool

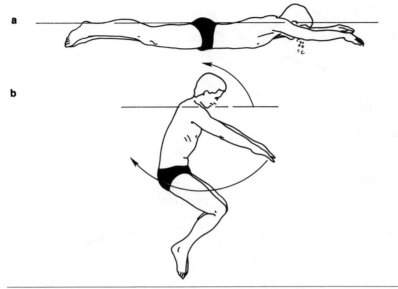

Figure 3.6. Prone float (a) with recovery to a stand (b).

wall, keeping your arms overhead and your elbows straight (see Figure 3.1). Flutter kick as you breath rhythmically: Inhale with your face turned to one side, then exhale with face in water.

Prone glide with flutter kick (five minutes): Flutter kick while holding onto kickboard.

Crawl armstroke while standing and then walking (five minutes).

Swim and/or water walk for a total of two minutes, resting as needed.

STEP 4

Rhythmic breathing review (four minutes). See Step 3.

Law of opposites (five minutes): Combine rhythmic breathing with the crawl hand motion, first while standing; then while walking; and then while swimming. When you turn your head during rhythmic breathing, the arm on the opposite side of your body is extended in front of you, while the arm on your breathing side is stretched behind you. As you turn your head back into the water, your arms switch positions (see Figures 3.7 and 3.8).

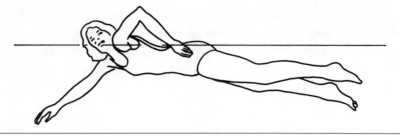

Figure 3.7. Crawl stroke.

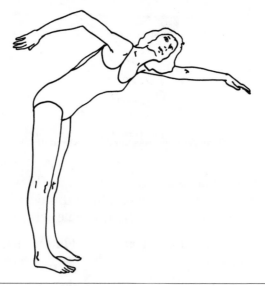

Figure 3.8. Law of opposites.

Overhand kickboard press (four minutes): Stand in chest-deep water. Grasp the edges of the kickboard that is floating in front of you; press the kickboard downward slowly and then slowly lift it back to the surface; repeat.

Swim for a total of three minutes, resting as needed.

STEP 5

Law of opposites review (three minutes). See Step 4.

Arm sculling exercise (five minutes): Stand in chest-deep water. Keeping your shoulders underwater, extend your arms out in front of you with your thumbs pointed downward. Sweep your arms outward keeping your pinkies up, then bring your arms back to the starting position keeping your thumbs up. The palms of your hands should face away from you as you press outward; as you bring your hands back inward, your palms should face inward (see Figure 3.9).

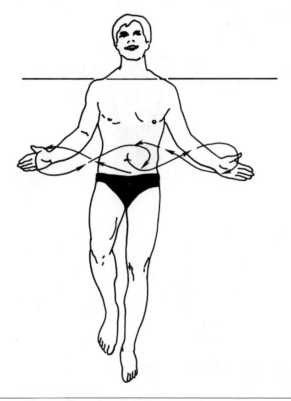

Figure 3.9. Treading water.

Treading (five minutes): Start in a standing position. Combine a wide sculling arm motion with a bicycle leg motion or scissors, frog, or flutter kick (see Figure 3.9). When practicing treading, begin in shallow water. If you are a new deep-water swimmer, practice by holding onto the edge of the pool with one hand. With practice, your strength, skill, efficiency, and confidence will let you tread in deep water without this assistance.

Swim for a total of four minutes, resting as needed.

STEP 6

Pendulum body swing (four minutes): Stand in neck-deep water. Hold on to the edge of the pool with both hands and keep your legs together with your body in a vertical position. Move your legs alternately to the right and to the left (see Figure 3.10).

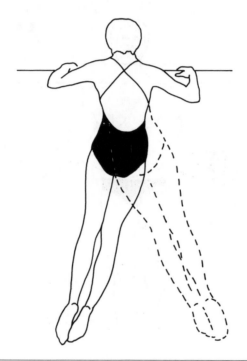

Figure 3.10. Pendulum body swing.

Back float recovery (four minutes): Assume a back float position (use a partner for support or use the pool's corner, if needed). Recover to a stand by piking (bending) at the waist, bending your knees, tucking your head forward, and scooping your arms downward behind you, and then in an upward motion, in order to stand (see Figure 3.11). Practice this several times.

Back flutter kick (four minutes): From a back float position, hold a kickboard on your stomach for support and kick.

Swim for a total of five minutes, resting as needed. Distance goal: 100 yards.

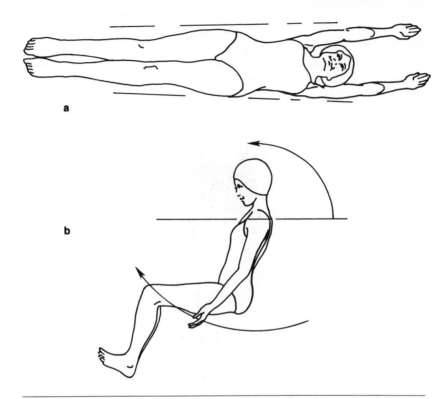

Figure 3.11. Back float recovery: from a supine float (a) to a stand (b).

STEP 7

Aqua skip exercise (four minutes): In waist-deep water, move your arms and legs as if you were skipping rope. Try it backwards as well as forward.

Leg lift exercise (four minutes): With your back against the pool wall, alternate lifting each leg toward the surface and lowering it to the pool's bottom. Try to keep your knees straight.

Sculling arm motion in back float position (three minutes): This is similar to the treading arm motion, but here you keep your hands close to your hips while pressing the water toward your body and then away from it. Flex your wrists, keeping fingertips up. Your hands will follow a figure-eight pattern (see Figure 3.12). You can add the flutter kick for better balance and propulsion.

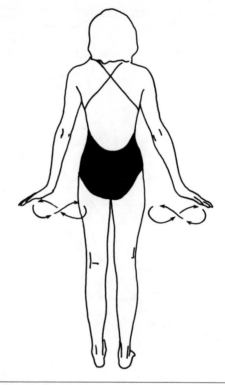

Figure 3.12. Sculling arm motion.

Swim for a total of seven minutes, resting as needed. Distance goal: 150 yards.

STEP 8

Aqua push ups (four minutes): Stand at the end of the pool and grasp the gutter with your hands shoulder's width apart. Bend your elbows and touch the edge of the pool with your chin. Then, straighten your elbows and lift yourself out of the water (see Figure 3.13). Do not lock your elbows.

Aqua sit ups (four minutes): With your back against the pool wall, hold on with your arms extended outward onto the deck and bring your heels to your buttocks while you draw your knees to your chest (see Figure 3.14).

Swim for a total of ten minutes, resting as needed. Distance goal: 200 yards.

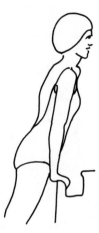

Figure 3.13. Aqua push up.

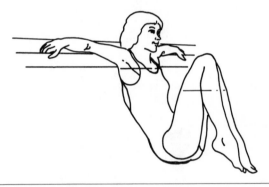

Figure 3.14. Aqua sit up.

Fartlek training: Try your ten-minute swim this way: Alternate your swimming speeds from slow to intermediate to fast. Monitor your heart rate to be sure you are staying within your THR range. Swim slowly when you need a rest period. Speed up again as you recover.

STEP 9

Open turn (two minutes): First walk and then swim to the wall with one of your arms extended (see Figure 3.15a). Grasp the edge and then bend your knees to your chest and place your feet on the wall in a push-off position (see Figure 3.15b). Bring both of your arms to an overhead position and push off the wall with your legs and glide (see Figure 3.15c).

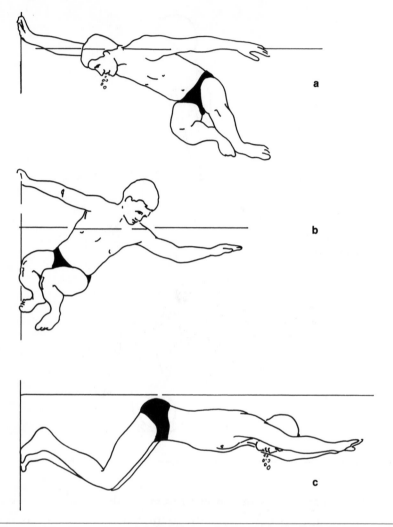

Figure 3.15. Open turn: (a) the approach; (b) the turn; and (c) the push-off.

Shoulder twist (two minutes): Stretch your arms outward and sideward at shoulder level under the water. Twist your shoulders, arms, and upper body to the right, keeping your feet in the same spot on the pool bottom. Alternate to the left.

Leg circles (two minutes): In a standing position, lift one leg from the bottom of the pool, keeping your knees straight, and circle your leg in both directions. Alternate with the other leg.

Swim for a total of twelve to fifteen minutes, resting as needed. Distance goal: 300 yards.

STEP 10

Aqua jumping jacks: In chest-deep water, bring your arms over head and move your feet apart. Then return to the starting position on the next jump with your feet together and your arms at your sides.

Static arm and leg stretches (see Step 1).

Swim for a total of twenty minutes, resting as needed. Distance goal: one-quarter mile (440 yards).

Suggestions for the quarter-mile swim: Mix the various types of swim equipment during your quarter-mile swim; for example, swim 100 yards using a kickboard, 100 yards with hand paddles, 100 yards with swim fins, and 100 yards with a pull-buoy.

Suggested Readings

By the author:

Swimming for Total Fitness: A Progressive Aerobic Program. (1981). Garden City, NY: Doubleday/Dolphin.

The W.E.T. Workout: Water Exercise Techniques to Help You Tone Up and Slim Down Aerobically. (1985). New York: Facts on File.

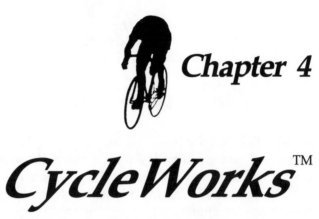

Chapter 4

CycleWorks™

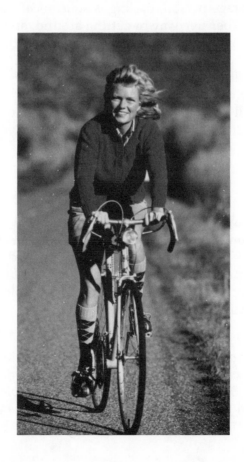

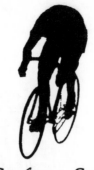

Go for a Spin

In July, 1986, for the first time, an American, Greg LeMond, won the world famous *Tour de France*. LeMond's accomplishment is a vivid reflection of the growth in popularity of cycling in the U.S. More than 75 million Americans cycle, making it one of our most popular sports.

For the average person, cycling is a means of transportation, a fun and inexpensive way of getting around, and a way to enjoy the outdoors. Biking also offers many fitness benefits including improved upper and lower body tone and improved aerobic fitness with little stress on the joints.

If your job or other daily commute allows you to travel by bicycle, you'll find that commuting by bike is a wonderful and convenient form of exercise. Perhaps for you, CycleWorks will become "Cycle-to-Work."

Gear Up

There are many models and types of bicycles available. If you have a basic one-speed bike, don't throw it out. It's perhaps one of the best two-wheeled fitness builders around. However, if you're in the market for a new bike, shop around for good quality within your price range. Consult a knowledgeable salesperson, a veteran cyclist, and/or *Consumer Reports*.

Types of Cycles
Your choice will depend on cost, use, and individual needs. A trip to the local bike shop will reveal a wide variety of bikes including 1-, 3-, 5-, 10-, 12-, 15-, and 18-speed bicycles. You'll probably find that the 1-, 3-, and 10-speed bikes are the most

common. The variety of styles and gear ratios includes the following:

High Riser. Designed for youngsters, it has twenty-inch or smaller wheels, a small frame, and a low center of gravity. High risers have anywhere from one to ten gears.

Middleweight. The middleweight includes a wide range of frame sizes, designs, and options. You sit upright. The tires are wider and the wheels usually have fenders (see Figure 4.1). There may be 1, 3, or 5 speeds.

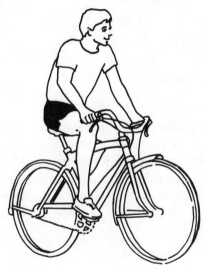

Figure 4.1. Middleweight/upright bicycle frame.

Racing/Touring. This is a lightweight bike with dropped handlebars, a narrow saddle, narrow tires, and no fenders (see Figure 4.2). They have 10, 12, 15, or 18 speeds.

City/Mountain/All-Terrain. This bike is designed for rugged terrain as well as city pavements. It can have as many as 18 gears.

Tri-Wheeler. These are adult tricycles which allow practical, comfortable transportation in a suburban environment.

Tandem. A two-person bicycle; the front rider controls the steering while both riders pedal.

Stationary. Stationary bikes are excellent for indoor exercise or for people who don't have access to quiet streets where cycling

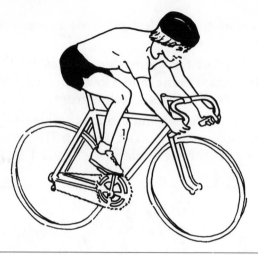

Figure 4.2. Racing frame.

is safe. Stationary bikes come in a variety of styles with several options, including adjustable resistance devices, arm-pumping handlebars, speedometers, odometers, and timers (see Figure 4.3). These cycles are unique because you can exercise privately, and they are also convenient for those with a busy schedule. With a stationary bike, you no longer need good weather for your CycleWorks.

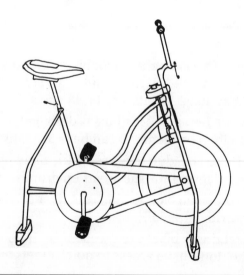

Figure 4.3. Stationary bicycle.

The Right Fit

Be sure to select the right size of bike frame. You have a choice of men's, women's, and *mixte* frames, all with standard sizes from nineteen to twenty-seven inches. A men's frame has a triangular shape. The horizontal top bar gives this frame the greatest strength and support. A woman's frame has a slanted top bar to allow women to ride in skirts. A *mixte* frame (Figure 4.4) has a top bar with less of a slant than that on a woman's bike, and therefore offers more support.

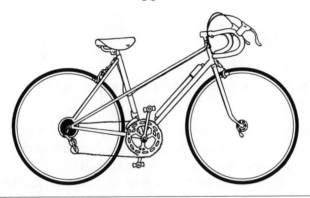

Figure 4.4. Mixte frame.

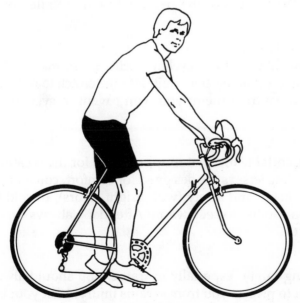

Figure 4.5. Determining proper fit is an important part of bicycle selection.

To determine your frame size, straddle a men's style bike with your feet flat on the floor. The frame should be one inch below your crotch. You should be able to sit comfortably on the seat and reach the gear controls and pedals. To gauge the proper fit when you're sitting in the saddle, push the pedal down to its lowest point; your knee should be slightly bent with your heel on the pedal (see Figure 4.5).

Seats come in various shapes and materials for both men and women. A good bike shop will help you make the necessary adjustments when you purchase a bike.

Dress Right

Wristwatch
Wear one to time your CycleWorks workout.

Shoes
A rubber-soled shoe with a good firm sole and a pair of socks are adequate for most riders. However, there are shoes with stiff soles that are designed for cycling to spread the resistance of the pedal over the entire foot to prevent foot fatigue. Cycling shoes for racing have cleats that grip the pedals so that the cyclist may use all 360 degrees of the pedal rotation to generate power.

Shorts
Comfortable slacks or shorts are fine for cycling. More serious cyclers might want to try cycling stretch shorts made out of Lycra. These have a chamois liner built into the crotch to reduce friction. Once you've tried them, you won't want to cycle in anything else.

Top
Any comfortable top that is appropriate for the weather is suitable. Cycling jerseys are designed for comfort, convenience (with back pockets), and safety (with bright colors). In cold weather, layer your clothes to keep warm. After dark, always wear a reflective vest.

Helmet
For riding safety, especially in traffic, you should always wear a helmet to protect you from serious injury. Visit your bike shop and try them on for comfort before you buy. Be sure that the helmet you choose meets safety standards.

Accessories

Mirrors
Rearview mirrors that attach to your helmet, bicycle, wrist, or glasses enable you to see behind without turning your head.

Gloves
Be sure there's sufficient padding on the palms, with fingertip openings for added comfort and mobility.

Goggles or Sunglasses
Wear some kind of eye protection to keep out dust. This is especially important if you wear contact lenses (wraparound glasses are best in this case).

Learn to Ride

If you don't already have a bike, borrow or rent one. When first learning to ride a bike, start with one that would normally be too small. Lower the seat so that when you are sitting your feet can easily reach the ground. Beginners should use upright handlebars for easier steering and a more comfortable body position. If possible, choose a bike with hand (caliper) rather than foot (coaster) brakes.

For your first riding lesson find an open, paved parking lot or park area. Choose a very slight incline; start your ride at the top.

1. Sit on the saddle with your feet easily touching the ground.
2. Grip both hand brakes to get the feel of stopping. Braking must be a conscious action; instinct often tells you to put your feet down to stop, but brakes are the only way to stop safely. For caliper brakes, usually the right brake controls the rear wheel and the left brake controls the front wheel. Apply brakes simultaneously. For coaster brakes, push the pedals backwards with your feet.
3. Keep your body weight centered on the saddle.
4. Look straight ahead rather than down at the front tire.
5. Keep your body relaxed, particularly your arms and shoulders, and breathe normally. The sooner you relax, the easier it will be to learn.

6. Use the handlebars to balance the bike. When the bike moves to the left, turn the handlebars to the right to compensate (and vice versa). This movement maintains your balance and keeps you traveling in a straight line. When first learning, don't worry if you are zigzagging; eventually your path will straighten out.
7. Keep your palms loose on the handgrips to allow for quick use of hand brakes.
8. Now you are ready to ride. Scoot the bike forward by shuffling your feet along the ground. It will be easy to move forward if you can roll down a slight hill and use your feet near the ground for balance.
9. After rolling down the incline, walk the bike back up the incline and try again.
10. As you gain balance and confidence, place one foot on a pedal, shuffling the other foot on the ground. Then try this with the other foot.
11. Take short breaks between rides to relax your tense muscles.
12. When you are ready to pedal, scoot the bike forward and place both feet on the pedals and coast. Begin pedaling slowly.
13. Once you have safely and confidently mastered these skills, you can raise the seat to a normal level. Your knee should be almost fully extended on the downward pedal, and you should be using calf muscles in addition to thigh muscles.

Gearing

Changing gears allows you to adapt pedaling power to the conditions opposing your forward motion (hills, wind, load, road surface, and fatigue). The goal is to keep your pedaling speed and effort as constant as possible.

On a three-speed bicycle, first gear is used for climbing hills, second gear is for riding on level ground, and third gear is for traveling downhill.

A ten-speed bike has a cluster of five gear sprockets at the rear wheel and two sprockets at the pedals; this cluster provides the ten positions or gears the chain can occupy. A ten-speed bike provides a greater number of gears that have the same purpose as the three-speed gears. There are two gear shift levers mounted

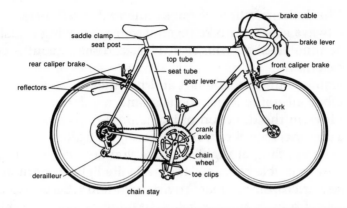

Figure 4.6. Typical five-speed bike.

on the frame or handlebars that control the two derailleurs. The right lever controls the rear derailleur; the left lever controls the front derailleur. The derailleurs move the chain from one sprocket to another, enabling you to move with more or less pedaling effort.

How to Change Gears

To change gears you must be pedaling. Anticipate changes in terrain and conditions, and change gears before pedaling becomes difficult. Shift before you start climbing a hill, and avoid getting caught in a high gear at a stoplight.

When changing gears, continue to pedal, but decrease foot pressure slightly and shift the lever. When shifting from a smaller to a larger sprocket, slow down the pedal action until the chain catches. After shifting, if there is a clattering sound, adjust the lever up or down slightly until the chain is fully engaged and operates quietly.

Safety Tips and Suggestions for CycleWorks

1. Check brakes by squeezing them when the bike is stationary. They should grip the wheel rims firmly in place. Check pads for excessive wear.
2. Check the tire pressure.

3. Check the position of the saddle and handlebars.
4. Always lock your bike (even if you are leaving it just for a minute). Ask you local bicycle dealer about bicycle insurance.
5. Know your hand signals and use them.
6. Obey all traffic signs, signals, and regulations.
7. Move in the direction of traffic flow.
8. Turn and look when maneuvering in traffic.
9. When cycling at night, be sure you are visible! In addition to visible clothing, have a white light in front and a red reflector in the rear. You can also add reflectors to your wheel spokes and pedals. A flashing beacon is good for additional visibility. Many municipal traffic laws require cyclists to wear reflective gear.
10. On bike paths, stay to the right and do not speed. Watch out for runners, pedestrians, and dogs.
11. Give pedestrians the right of way. Avoid sidewalks.
12. Dress according to the weather.
13. Tote belongings comfortably and safely. Wear clothing with pockets or use a knapsack, saddlebag, or bicycle basket(s).
14. Carry a pump, repair kit, and water bottle for longer rides.
15. Remember to check your pulse periodically to be sure you are in your THR range.

10
STEP
Progressive CycleWorks Program

The following CycleWorks program is a 10-step progression. Start with the step that matches your fitness level. Once you are comfortable with that activity level, progress to the next step. This program can be modified for use with a stationary bike as well. Measure your distance with an odometer and simulate hills by periodically adjusting resistance. Always perform a warm-up and a cool-down as a part of your CycleWorks.

Before beginning this program, review the elements of riding: starting and stopping, riding a straight line, and changing direction.

STEP 1

Ride on flat terrain where there is no traffic. Cycle continuously for five minutes. Coast one minute and repeat three times.

STEP 2

Cycle continuously on flat terrain for ten minutes. Coast for one minute and repeat.

STEP 3

Cycle continuously for twenty minutes. Measure and record the distance you cover.

STEP 4

Cycle on slightly hilly terrain for twenty minutes. Change gears as needed.

STEP 5

Cycle moderately for five minutes, then vigorously for two minutes. Repeat this three times.

STEP 6

Cycle for twenty minutes in three six-minute sets. For each set, begin *slowly* and gradually increase to your maximum speed. Even at you maximum speed, you should still be capable of carrying on a conversation. Coast for one minute after each set.

STEP 7

Cycle for twenty minutes at a steady brisk pace. Increase mileage from Step 3.

STEP 8

Cycle in two ten-minute *fartlek* sets. Do this by beginning slowly and progressing to moderate and then full speed within five minutes. Coast one minute and repeat *fartlek* set.

STEP 9

Cycle continuously for twenty minutes on hilly terrain at medium intensity. Change gears when necessary.

STEP 10

Cycle continuously for twenty minutes and measure the distance you cover. (Use an odometer, if possible.) Try to increase the distance you cover in twenty minutes as you progress in your CycleWorks program.

Chapter 5

NutritionWorks™

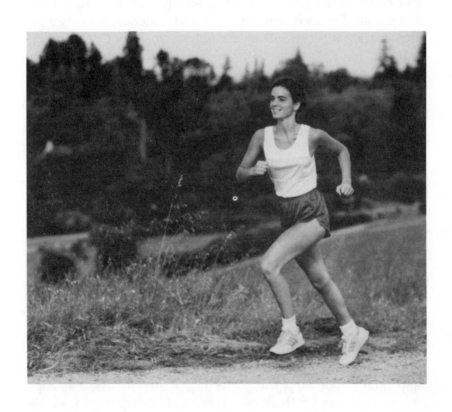

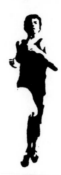

The Health Twins

The health twins are proper nutrition and exercise. There is a definite relationship between proper nutrition and fitness; that is why you need both NutritionWorks and FitnessWorks working for you! Table 5.1 summarizes the role of the seven nutrients your body needs. The first three (carbohydrates, protein, and fat) are called the macronutrients, which form the bulk of our food intake. The next two (vitamins and minerals) are called the micronutrients because they are only a small (but very important) part of our food intake. The last two (fiber and water) are sometimes not listed as nutrients but they are essential for keeping us going. All seven of the food components are necessary for our health and activity.

In the opinion of medical and nutritional authorities (such as the American Heart Association, the American Dietetic Association, and the National Cancer Institute), Americans can reduce their risk of serious health problems by adopting a diet that is low in fat, high in complex carbohydrates, and moderate in protein. Table 5.2 compares the NutritionWorks recommendation for healthy individuals with the dietary pattern many Americans now consume.

The percentages in Table 5.2 are by calories, which are units of energy. A gram is a unit of mass—a level teaspoon of most food substances is about five grams. Both carbohydrates and protein contain four calories per gram, whereas fat contains nine calories per gram.

Tables 5.3 and 5.4 compare the calculations of caloric percentages for daily intake following the NutritionWorks pattern and daily intake following the pattern of many Americans. Each sample day totals 1,500 calories. These tables illustrate that a well-balanced diet involves more than counting calories.

Table 5.1 Summary of the Seven Nutrients

Nutrient	Function of Nutrient in Body	Ordinary Food Sources for Nutrient
Carbohydrates	Main source of fuel that supplies energy for body functioning, heat, and activity; the ratio of complex to simple carbohydrates in the diet should be 5 to 1	There are two kinds: 1. Simple carbohydrates—*all* sugars 2. Complex carbohydrates—beans, potatoes, yams, and whole grains like bread, rice, pasta, cereals
Protein	Required for growth, maintenance, and repair of all body tissues; also used to supply energy	Meat, poultry, fish, dairy products, peas, beans, grains
Fat	Stored energy to be used under emergency conditions; supports the internal organs; gives the body its contour	Butter, margarine, meat, poultry, fish, dairy products
Vitamins	They are not energy nutrients themselves but they are constituents of body enzymes, which are chemicals required for the metabolism of the three energy nutrients	Most foods. There are two classes: 1. Water soluble (B and C) found in fruits, vegetables, whole grains, meats, and dairy products 2. Fat soluble (A, D, and E) found in meat, poultry, fish, dairy products, and dark green or yellow vegetables. Vitamin K is fat soluble and is synthesized in the body

(Cont.)

Table 5.1 (Cont.)

Nutrient	Function of Nutrient in Body	Ordinary Food Sources for Nutrient
Minerals	Inorganic chemicals that are either constituents of the body structures (bones, teeth, muscles, nerves, and blood) or are required in small amounts for chemical reactions of the body	Most foods contain some minerals. Some foods are known to be especially good sources of certain essential minerals; for example, milk products are a good source of calcium. Some minerals are only required in exceedingly small amounts; for example, iodine from sea foods.
Fiber	Nondigestible carbohydrates which influence the speed with which the other nutrients move through the digestive system	Whole grains, fresh fruits and vegetables, bran (the protective outer covering of the kernel of wheat, oats, or corn)
Water	Component of body fluids and tissues; provides the medium in which most of the body's chemical reactions occur	Tap water, beverages, fruits, and vegetables

Table 5.2 Typical and Recommended Dietary Patterns (% of Daily Calories)

	NutritionWorks Pattern		Pattern of Many Americans	
	Recommended	Range	Average	Range
Carbohydrate	70%	60%–80%	30%	20%–40%
Protein	15%	15%–20%	25%	20%–30%
Fat	15%	10%–20%	45%	40%–50%
	100%		100%	

Table 5.3 Typical NutritionWorks Daily Intake (Calculated for 1,500 Calories)

Carbohydrates	262.5	grams × 4 calories/gram =	1,050 calories
Protein	56.25	grams × 4 calories/gram =	225 calories
Fat	25	grams × 9 calories/gram =	225 calories
		Total =	1,500 calories

Calculating the Percentages

Carbohydrates $\dfrac{1{,}050 \text{ calories}}{1{,}500 \text{ (total calories)}} \times 100 = 70\%$

Protein $\dfrac{225 \text{ calories}}{1{,}500 \text{ (total calories)}} \times 100 = 15\%$

Fat $\dfrac{225 \text{ calories}}{1{,}500 \text{ (total calories)}} \times 100 = 15\%$

Table 5.4 Pattern of Many Americans' Daily Intake (Calculated for 1,500 Calories)

Carbohydrates	112.5 grams × 4 calories/gram =	450 calories
Protein	93.7 grams × 4 calories/gram =	375 calories
Fat	75 grams × 9 calories/gram =	675 calories
	Total =	1,500 calories

Calculating the Percentages

Carbohydrates $\dfrac{450 \text{ calories}}{1{,}500 \text{ (total calories)}} \times 100 = 30\%$

Protein $\dfrac{375 \text{ calories}}{1{,}500 \text{ (total calories)}} \times 100 = 25\%$

Fat $\dfrac{675 \text{ calories}}{1{,}500 \text{ (total calories)}} \times 100 = 45\%$

By following the NutritionWorks pattern, you will have a healthy and balanced diet. The NutritionWorks balance for healthy living lowers your fat intake, increases consumption of complex carbohydrates and fiber, and moderates your protein intake (see the MenuWorks section for how to accomplish this).

Exercise, Weight Loss, and Calories

Approximately 65 million Americans are on a diet at any one time. Yet dieting alone rarely results in significant or permanent weight loss. Many popular diets require cutting calories below a level that is safe or balanced nutritionally. You should combine diet *and* exercise to be successful in losing and maintaining a desired weight.

Exercising can actually make dieting easier. Current research suggests that moderate exercise will temporarily reduce your appetite. Another bonus of exercise is that it raises your metabolism so that you continue to burn calories at a higher than normal rate following exercise.

The safest and most effective way to lose weight is to do so gradually. Up to two pounds of weight loss per week is considered safe. If you wish to lose weight, you can calculate how many calories to cut from your diet. However, your daily intake should never drop below 1,200 calories. One pound of fat yields approximately 3,500 calories. To lose one pound of fat a week by dieting alone you would need to cut 500 calories a day from your diet. If you combine regular exercise with reduced caloric intake, more calories will be burned. For example, by burning 500 calories a day through exercise, another pound could be lost each week. Thus through diet and exercise you could lose two pounds per week.

Caloric expenditure during exercise depends on the intensity of the exercise and your body weight. More calories are burned at higher intensities and body weights. You can calculate the approximate caloric expenditure of your exercise by looking at Table 5.5. Note that a moderate intensity is most effective for weight control and maintenance. This is because primarily fat is burned during moderate exercise; also it is possible to exercise longer at this pace. Carbohydrate is the primary energy source used at high work levels, and it is also not possible to maintain such a pace for more than a few minutes.

Table 5.5 Physical Activity and Caloric Expenditure*

Work Intensity	Heart Rate	Calories/ Minute	Activities
Light	Below 120	Under 5	Walking, golf, bowling, volleyball, most forms of work
Moderate**	120 to 150	5 to 10	Jogging, tennis, cycling, hiking, aerobic dance, racquetball, strenuous work, basketball
Heavy	Above 150	Above 10	Running, fast swimming, other brief intense efforts

*Values are for person weighing approximately 150 pounds. Add 10% for every 15 pounds above this weight; for every 15 pounds below 150, subtract 10%.
**Preferred pace for weight control benefits.
Note. From *Physiology of Fitness*, 2nd Ed., (p. 88) by Brian J. Sharkey, 1984, Champaign, IL: Human Kinetics Publishers, Inc. Copyright 1984 by Brian J. Sharkey. Reprinted with permission.

Though metabolism depends on a variety of factors (age, activity level, weight, etc.), you can determine the approximate number of calories needed to maintain a desired weight. Merely multiply the desired weight by 15 (if you are over twenty-one). For example, if your desired weight is 120 pounds, your daily caloric intake would be approximately 1,800 calories. This figure can then be used as a general guide when planning your NutritionWorks and FitnessWorks goals for maintaining a specific weight.

Benefits of Following NutritionWorks

Eating NutritionWorks foods will give you a sense of well-being and help you maintain your desirable weight. However, these aren't the only benefits. Recent research indicates that diets high in complex carbohydrates and fiber and low in fat and cholesterol can help reduce your chance of heart disease and certain types of cancer. Decreasing your salt intake helps to reduce your risk of hypertension. So, follow NutritionWorks for good health.

NutritionWorks Goals

1. Limit intake of total fat and cholesterol.
2. Limit sodium (salt) intake.
3. Avoid simple sugars; increase intake of complex carbo-hydrates and fiber.

The following lists give you suggestions for meeting the NutritionWorks goals, indicating which foods you should eat and which foods you should limit or avoid. Note that these lists are not exhaustive.

1. *Limit intake of total fat and cholesterol.*

NutritionWorks Foods	Foods to Avoid or Limit
Lean Meats	Fried foods
Skim and low-fat milk and other dairy products	Cooking oil
	Butter
Poultry (without skin)	Margarine
Fish	Salad dressings
Fresh fruits	Mayonnaise
Fresh vegetables	Fatty red meats
No-oil salad dressings	Cold cuts/lunch meats
Breads prepared without oils or shortening	Hot dogs
	Sausage
Tuna fish in water	Egg yolks
Egg whites	Cookies
	Chicken skins
	Tuna fish in oil
	Heavy cream
	Half-and-Half
	Whole milk
	Whole milk cheeses

2. *Limit sodium (salt) intake.* Dairy products and meats contain a significant amount of sodium naturally. However, they are acceptable and advocated when consumed in moderate quantities. The NutritionWorks program will

provide enough sodium in the diet to meet most individuals' needs. You can eliminate the use of table salt and
still meet sodium requirements.

NutritionWorks Foods	Foods to Avoid or Limit
Fresh fruits and vegetables	Salt—when cooking
Unsalted cheese	Potato chips, pretzels, salted crackers, salted nuts
Hot cereals prepared without salt	
Breads (low salt)	Canned foods (unless unsalted)
Natural/no-salt peanut butter	Hot dogs
Rice cakes	Bacon
Unsalted crackers	Ham, lunch meats
Low-fat unsalted cheese	Dry cereals (except no-salt varieties)
	Olives and pickles
	Cheese (except no-salt varieties)
	Commercial peanut butter

3. *Avoid simple sugars; increase intake of complex carbohydrates
   and fiber.*

NutritionWorks Foods	Foods to Avoid or Limit
Fruit juices without added sugar	Table sugar, corn syrup
Preserves prepared without sugar	Cookies
Fresh fruits and vegetables	Cakes and pastry
Frozen vegetables	Soda
Unsweetened canned and jarred fruits	Pancake syrup
	Candied fruits
Unsweetened frozen fruits	Jelly, preserves, and jam
Whole grain bread	Candy
Brown rice	Sweetened dry cereals
Whole grain cereals, oatmeal	Prepared cake mixes
Wheat and rice cakes	White breads
Bran	Canned fruits in heavy syrup
Plain nonfat or low-fat yogurt	Yogurts prepared with sugar or corn syrup
Beans, all types (unsalted)	

NutritionWorks Tips

1. Prepare foods without added oils or fats. Foods cooked with added oil may taste good, but they don't wear well!
2. Trim all meat, fish, or poultry of any visible fat or skin. Select lean cuts of meat.
3. Roast, bake, broil, boil, or microwave foods instead of frying or barbecuing.
4. Use fresh instead of processed foods.
5. Select skim or low-fat milk (1 percent fat) and dairy products.
6. Limit cholesterol by eating no more than three egg yolks per week. Egg whites contain no cholesterol and need not be limited.
7. Limit meats to about four ounces at any one meal and six ounces total per day.
8. Use herbs, spices, or lemon juice for food flavoring instead of salt.
9. Steam fresh or frozen vegetables to preserve vitamins. Avoid overcooking.
10. Save yourself extra cooking time by preparing larger quantities, especially entrees, which can be frozen or refrigerated for future use.
11. Prepare brown rice ahead of time so that it is always on hand.
12. Use bananas, berries, or raisins as sweeteners on cereal and in yogurt or for snacks.
13. Make your own beef or chicken stock for soups by placing the drippings of these cooked foods in the refrigerator (not the freezer). The fat can then be easily removed. Store homemade stock in refrigerator or freezer for future use.
14. Read labels carefully. The major ingredient is listed first. The next ingredient contains the next largest quantity, and so forth.
15. Drink coffee in moderation.
16. Always eat a breakfast that is high in complex carbohydrates, which supply the energy needed to face the day's activities. Oatmeal and shredded wheat are good sources of complex carbohydrates.
17. Drink alcohol in moderation if you desire. A glass of wine with lunch or dinner certainly won't ruin everything!

18. Look for jams, jellies, preserves, and conserves that are prepared with fruit and fruit juices only.
19. Limit or avoid regular sodas, which contain too much sugar. Also avoid Club soda which contains salt. Drink seltzer or water. Add seltzer to fruit juices to create your own natural sodas.
20. Don't assume that the word *natural* on food packaging means that you're getting a good thing. Read the ingredients carefully.
21. Beware of other names for sugar: fructose (fruit sugar), corn syrup, and sucrose.
22. Prepare raw vegetables for snacks. Try carrots, celery, cherry tomatoes, and cucumbers.
23. Avoid food shopping when you're hungry. You may be unable to resist the lure of chocolate chip cookies or cheesecake.
24. You don't necessarily have to shop in a health food store. The ordinary supermarket can be your headquarters for some of the most healthful foods around.
25. If you eat out frequently, follow these additional Nutrition-Works Guidelines:

    - Ask for sauces and salad dressing "on the side" or order salad with no dressing.
    - Order nonalcoholic drinks, particularly those with fruit juices and seltzer, and water.
    - Don't eat everything on your plate if you're full. Don't be shy about asking for a doggie bag. Leftovers make quick meals the next day.
    - Order baked potatoes (without butter or sour cream) instead of french fries or home fries.
    - Ask that your food be prepared without oils, sauces, salt, or MSG.
    - Avoid fast food chains unless you're hitting the salad bar.
    - Order poultry and fish instead of red meats. Keep the main portion small to medium (three to six ounces).

MenuWorks

The following are two samples of daily menus; these should give you an idea of how you can apply the principles of Nutrition-

Works to your life-style. "Menu A" is based on breakfast at home, a brown-bag lunch, and a home-cooked dinner. "Menu B" is based on breakfast at home and lunch and dinner in restaurants.

Menu A

```
Calories: approx. 1500
Carbohydrates: approx. 70%
Protein: approx. 20%
Fat: approx. 10%
```

Breakfast: Orange juice

Oatmeal with bran and low-fat milk, sweetened with banana slices (or raisins)

Slice of whole-grain bread toasted with fruit-only conserve

Postum, Decaf, or coffee with low-fat milk

Lunch: Tuna fish on two slices whole grain bread

(brown bag)   Fresh veggie sticks (celery and carrot sticks)

Chilled baked potato

Fresh fruit

Dinner: *Appetizer:*

(at home)   Serving of canteloupe

Entree:

Fish broiled (in small amount of water). (Do *not* turn fish when broiling.) Served with brown rice, tossed salad, homemade apple-sauce, and fresh or frozen broccoli

Dessert:

Instant blueberry cheesecake. Place one slice of whole grain raisin bread on a plate. Spread with a layer of fruit-only conserve, to desired taste. On top of this spread a generous layer of low-fat (1%), no-salt cottage cheese. Sprinkle with cinnamon. If desired, add a layer of blueberries, strawberries, sliced banana, or any other fruit in season.

Beverage (juice or skim milk)

Evening   Fresh fruit and/or rice cakes with fruit-only
snack: conserve.

Menu B

> Calories: approx. 1500
> Carbohydrates: approx. 65%
> Protein: approx. 20%
> Fat: approx. 15%

Breakfast: Grapefruit juice
                   Shredded wheat with low-fat milk, sweetened
                   with banana slices, raisins, or other fruit
                   Whole grain raisin bread with fruit-only con-
                   serve or peanut butter (no-salt, no-sugar
                   variety)
                   Herb tea

Lunch: Sliced white meat turkey or roast beef on rye
(restaurant)   or whole wheat bread with lettuce and tomato.
                   Hold the salt and mayonnaise.
                   Fresh fruit salad
                   Beverage

Dinner: Vegetable soup
(restaurant)   Tossed salad
                   Bread
                   Roast quarter chicken, skin removed
                   Baked potato
                   Green vegetable
                   Beverage (white wine, juice)
                   Dessert:
                   Fresh fruit cup
                   Hot beverage

Evening   Apple butter on rice cakes or instant rice
snack: pudding. Place desired amount cooked brown
                   rice in a dessert dish. Mix with raisins to
                   desired sweetness. Add low-fat (1%) milk to
                   obtain desired consistency. Sprinkle with cin-
                   namon. Serve warm or cold.

The NutritionWorks Program

The following are ten highlights of NutritionWorks.

1. Begin the program with foods on the list that you already like; add new foods as you begin to assume your new NutritionWorks life-style.
2. Eat a variety of foods from the four basic food groups:
   - Meats or meat alternatives (lean): one or more servings, totaling three to six ounces daily.
   - Dairy products (skim or low-fat): two to four cups daily.
   - Fruits and vegetables: four or more three-ounce servings. Include a deep yellow or dark green vegetable daily. Include a citrus fruit (or juice) daily.
   - Grains: four or more servings daily (one slice of bread is a serving).
3. Plan your meals and snacks to fit into your schedule and to avoid hunger.
4. Include complex carbohydrates (starches) in all your meals (bread, rice, barley, cereals, potatoes, yams, vegetables). Eat whole grains frequently. Remember, starches are good for you.
5. Include a high-protein food at all or most meals (meats, dairy products, or complementary protein combination). However, it is not necessary to consume large amounts of protein.
6. Eat red meats three or fewer times per week. Choose poultry or fish for main entrees.
7. Prepare food without fats or oils. Limit or avoid prepared high-fat foods.
8. Keep sugar and other simple carbohydrates to a minimum.
9. Snack on fresh fruits, vegetables, and no-salt carbohydrates.
10. Avoid overeating; eat slowly and stop when you're satisfied.

CookWorks

The following are gourmet CookWorks for those days when you want to prepare a home-cooked meal.

Sole Hawaiian (serves 4-6)

     1 red onion, sliced
     1 red pepper, sliced
     1 banana, thinly sliced
     1 mango, sliced (after slicing, squeeze remaining mango for juice and save)
     1 12-ounce can of unsweetened pineapple juice concentrate
     1 teaspoon soy sauce (low-sodium)
     1 tablespoon white wine
     1/2 teaspoon lemon juice
     1/2 teaspoon lemon peel
     1/2 teaspoon ginger, freshly grated
     1 pound of sole filet
     2 teaspoons arrowroot or cornstarch

Microwave onion and red pepper for 2 minutes, or boil for 3-5 minutes, depending on preferred tenderness of vegetable.

Gently mix together banana, mango with juice, and 6 ounces of pineapple juice and set aside in small bowl. Divide mixture in half. Set aside one half to be used for the sauce.

Marinade

In large bowl pour in 6 remaining ounces of pineapple juice. Add soy sauce, wine, lemon juice, lemon peel, and ginger.

Place fish in marinade and let sit for 15 minutes. Place marinated fish in foil-lined baking dish. Combine red pepper, onion, and half of banana/mango mixture. Place the mixture on fish. Fold foil by pinching foil together. This will prevent fish from drying out. Bake 20 minutes at 350° F. Fish may need more or less baking time, depending on thickness of fillet. Check after 15 minutes with a fork. Fish will flake when done.

Sauce

Bring the other half of the fruit mixture to boil over medium heat. Quickly add arrowroot. Turn heat down when sauce thickens. Place fish on a platter and garnish with sauce. Serve with brown rice.

Preparation time: 30-40 minutes

Baked Stuffed Chicken (serves 6)

     3 cups cooked brown rice (approx. 1 cup uncooked)
     3-4 slices of fresh ginger
     1 cup dried mixed fruit, diced
     1/2 cup of currants
     6 chicken breast cutlets (skinless)
     1/4 cup white wine

> 2 pears, thinly sliced
> 1 6-ounce can of unthawed, unsweetened pineapple juice concentrate
> 2 teaspoons cornstarch or arrowroot

Step 1

Add ginger to rice and prepare according to package directions, but add no salt. Remove ginger from cooked rice and discard.

Step 2

In a bowl mix currants with diced fruit. Sprinkle water over fruit and microwave on High for 2 minutes or boil for 5 minutes. Drain remaining fruit juice and discard. Fold fruit mixture into cooked rice.

Step 3

Spoon fruit-rice mixture in center of each chicken breast filet. Roll up. Place fold face down in baking dish. Add wine. Bake in oven at 350° for approximately 10 minutes with cover on; then another 10 minutes with cover off, basting occasionally to keep the chicken moist. During the last few minutes of cooking, place pears over the chicken. Prepare sauce.

Step 4

Pineapple Sauce

In a saucepan bring pineapple juice to boil. Add cornstarch and stir vigorously for 2 minutes or until it thickens. Once thickened, turn heat immediately to low. Pour pineapple sauce over baked chicken and serve.

Preparation time using microwaved brown rice: 45 minutes

Preparation time cooking brown rice on stove: 1 hour and 15 minutes.

Creamy Velvet Chiffon Cheese Pudding (makes 2 9-inch pies)

> 1-1/2 pints of low-fat, low-salt cottage cheese
> 8 ounces of hoop cheese or low-salt farmer cheese
> 18 ounces of undiluted frozen apple juice concentrate, thawed
> 3 packets of unflavored gelatin
> 1 teaspoon vanilla
> 3 egg whites
> 1/2 teaspoon grated lemon
> 1/2 teaspoon lemon juice

Place the cheeses in a bowl and beat until smooth (about 3 minutes). Boil apple juice. Remove from heat and add the gelatin slowly, stirring until it's dissolved. Add the cheese and vanilla to the juice mixture. Beat the egg whites separately until stiff peaks form. Fold into gelatin mixture. Pour cheese mixture into piecrusts (recipe follows) or into a pudding mold. Chill until set (1 hour if frozen, 2 hours if refrigerated).

Toppings (optional)

Spread strawberry or blueberry conserve over pie. Or, place 1 cup of fresh blueberries or sliced strawberries on top of pie.

Note: For optimum results, allow pudding to set by chilling in freezer for one hour or in the refrigerator for several hours before adding the topping.

Preparation time: approximately 30 minutes (allow approximately 3 hours for chilling)

Piecrust for No-Bake Dessert

> 3 cups oatmeal (not instant)
> 1/2 cup raisins
> 1 cup thawed apple juice concentrate

Place oatmeal in two pie pans, spreading out evenly. Bake at 350° for 15 minutes. Remove from oven and add raisins. Pour 1/2 cup of apple juice concentrate into each pie pan. Mix well. Spread mixture evenly on bottom and side of pans. Bake again at 350° for 10 minutes. Allow to cool.

Pumpkin-Chiffon Pie (makes 2 9-inch pies)

> 2 cups canned pumpkin
> 1/2 to 1 cup date sugar to taste
> 6 egg whites, lightly beaten
> 2 cups evaporated low-fat skimmed milk
> 1 teaspoon vanilla
> 1 teaspoon cinnamon
> 1/2 teaspoon ground ginger
> 1/2 teaspoon nutmeg

Combine the pumpkin, date sugar, egg whites, evaporated milk, vanilla, and spices. Beat or blend until smooth. Pour into piecrust (recipe follows). Bake at 375° for 30-35 minutes or until pumpkin is set. Allow to cool and then freeze for one hour.

Preparation time: approximately 1 hour (allow approximately 3 hours for chilling)

Piecrust for Baked Dessert

3 cups of oatmeal (not instant)
1/2 cup raisins
1 cup thawed apple juice concentrate

Mix ingredients and divide evenly into two pie pans. Press mixture uniformly onto bottom and sides of pans. Pour pumpkin mixture into pans. Bake according to pie filling directions.

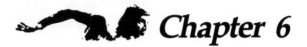

Chapter 6

FitnessWorks™
Q's and A's

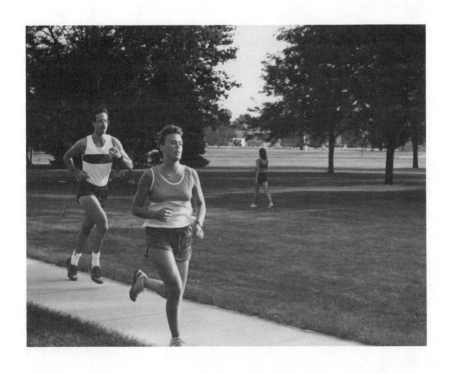

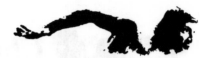

This chapter answers questions that many people ask once they decide to start an exercise program. The chapter is organized by topic, starting with general training, and moving on to the specific FitnessWorks activities, followed by questions on safety, beauty, and nutrition. It is likely the questions you have concerning your own FitnessWorks will be answered in these pages.

TrainingWorks

Question

I've never been involved in a sports or exercise program, but vigorous workouts do not appeal to me. Is it possible to get any aerobic effect from a slow, easy workout?

Answer

Yes. Current research is indicating that moderate, slow exercise can be very beneficial for your health, including your cardiovascular system. Try to build up your exercise program to at least thirty minutes a session, three times a week. Consistency is the key.

Question

How much and how often should I exercise to maintain fitness?

Answer

Follow the recommended guidelines from your FitnessWorks F.I.T. principle:

- F = Frequency—exercise for a minimum of three times per week (if possible, five is best)

- I = Intensity—exercise at your target heart rate (approximately 75 percent of your maximum heart rate) during your main set
- T = Time—the duration of your workout can vary from thirty minutes to one hour; however, your main aerobic set should be at least twenty minutes in length, with at least a five-minute warm-up and a five-minute cool down.

Question

Isn't all exercise good for your heart and lungs?

Answer

Not necessarily. You might enjoy a particular activity, but only a regular, sustained exercise program, which includes an aerobic activity such as brisk walking, jogging, swimming or cycling, will improve your cardiovascular system and burn off calories. Anaerobic activities (e.g. weight lifting) may give other benefits such as strength but will not provide you with cardiovascular fitness.

Question

Will I be tired after I exercise?

Answer

At times you may be tired. It depends on your application of the F.I.T. principle—the frequency, intensity and duration of your workouts. Most likely, exercise will stimulate your body. You will feel more relaxed and look better. If you exercise before going to work, you'll discover that your workout may give you more energy than you had before. If you exercise in the evening hours, leave ample time to unwind and relax before bedtime.

Question

Why is a lower resting heart rate better than a higher one?

Answer

A physically fit person's heart rate is usually somewhat slower because it has become stronger and more efficient. A heart that beats slowly doesn't have to work as hard to pump blood.

Question

How should I breathe when exercising?

Answer

Your basic breathing technique is to inhale and exhale continuously, never holding your breath.

Question

What are the signs and symptoms of overtraining?

Answer

Overtraining is similar to the word *burnout* often used in the work setting. You can also burn out on exercise. Here are some common symptoms of overtraining:

1. Excessive fatigue after an average workout
2. Lack of enthusiasm about your next session
3. Difficulty sleeping
4. Lack of energy
5. High morning pulse rate
6. Uncontrollable appetite or no appetite at all
7. Miscellaneous aches and pains

If you consistently experience one or more of these symptoms, you are overtraining. You can treat this trend by listening to your body. If you really don't feel like exercising, then take a break. After a couple of days, return to your FitnessWorks, but with less intensity. Try alternating days off with days of exercise. Your body needs anywhere from twenty-four to forty-eight hours of rest to recover from strenuous workouts. Warm baths, massages, and saunas pamper your body and help it to heal itself. You should always listen to your body. If you find that you continually overtrain, you might try a less taxing sports activity.

Question

How do I know if I'm working hard enough?

Answer

Your workout should bring on a degree of exhilaration, but not exhaustion to the point of gasping. You must exercise hard enough to elevate your heart rate to your THR (target heart rate) as described in chapter 1. If you are so short of breath that you cannot carry on a conversation at the same time, you are probably working too hard.

Question

I am almost sixty years old. Can I learn new fitness skills at this age?

Answer

Certainly! All it takes is a positive attitude and a progressive training program. FitnessWorks skills are lifetime sports activities. Senior and Masters competitions include adult groupings from twenty-five to ninety and above.

Question

Since the passing of Jim Fixx, the noted running enthusiast who suffered a heart attack while jogging, there has been talk recently about exercise-induced deaths. Shouldn't regular exercise prevent heart attacks?

Answer

Jim Fixx had an underlying heart condition that was genetic; his father also died at a young age from a heart attack. The question remains: Did regular running prolong his life? We will never really know for certain. There is also no definitive answer to the question of whether exercise prevents heart attacks. There are too many variables in the issue of heart attack and exercise. A moderate amount of brisk exercise may lessen a person's chances of having a heart attack. However, people who suffer from obesity, high blood pressure, or heart problems should have a physical checkup and follow their doctor's recommendations before starting an exercise program. In addition to exercise, current research is revealing that diet plays an important role in the incidence of heart disease. A moderate exercise program and a well-balanced diet are safe bets for lowering your risk of heart disease.

Question

Can FitnessWorks help me cope with stress?

Answer

People find many ways to cope with stress; unfortunately many choose unhealthy methods: smoking, drugs, overeating, or habitual drinking. Many people find that exercising is a better and healthier alternative for coping with stress and making life-style changes.

Question

Will exercise negate the harmful effects of smoking?

Answer

Unfortunately, whether they exercise or not, smokers run a higher health risk than nonsmokers of developing lung cancer, heart disease, and emphysema. Many smokers find it more difficult to exercise than nonsmokers. Conclusive research from the Surgeon General shows that smoking is harmful to your health. As you progress in your FitnessWorks program, you will find it easier to exercise if you eliminate your smoking habit.

Question

Is it possible to reapportion my body?

Answer

Reapportioning your body often means a redistribution of your body's weight. Since muscle weighs more than fat, exercise may actually increase your body weight at the same time it decreases the amount of fat in your body. You may look thinner even if your body weight remains similar.

The FitnessWorks program will help you tone up and lose weight. However, it is very difficult to change the body proportions that you were born with. Only through your FitnessWorks activities can you effectively burn up fat and build up muscle tone.

Question

I am interested in developing my FitnessWorks to participate in a triathlon. Where can I go for more information?

Answer

There are several how-to books on this subject. Check your local bookstore. In addition, most newsstands carry triathlon magazines as well as those devoted to swimming, cycling, running, and walking, which provide you with triathlon information.

SportsWorks

Question

What is low-impact aerobics?

Answer

Low-impact refers to the reduced jarring effects of sports activities on your joints. The low-impact aerobic activities highlighted in FitnessWorks are swimming, walking, and cycling. A higher impact aerobic activity is jogging. Low- or no-impact activities are appropriate for people who have joint problems, are overweight, or have other conditions which require non-jarring motion.

Question

What is a "runner's high"?

Answer

It is a euphoric feeling that occurs in most aerobic activities when your body is warmed up. You may experience a feeling of exhilaration and calmness, and you seem to have limitless energy. This feeling also can be described as a "second wind." During this high, your body is producing endorphins, chemicals which may contribute to this sensation.

Question

Are weights helpful in increasing the intensity of my FootWorks?

Answer

Ankle, hand-held, and wrist weights can be used when walking or jogging to increase aerobic stress and upper body strength. However, if you have joint problems or hypertension, refrain from their use.

Question

I don't know how to swim. What simple exercise can I begin with in the water?

Answer

The most basic exercise is to water walk. Many pools have shallow water, and you can even hold on to the edge for balance. Slowly increase your pace to a jog.

Question

What's aqua jogging and how do I do it?

Answer

Aqua jogging is the same as dry land jogging. Although it provides all of the cardiovascular benefits of regular jogging, it is easier on your joints and is a form of no-impact aerobics. Do aqua jogging in any water depth. When jogging in deep water, use a flotation vest. An arm-pumping motion will give added aerobic benefits. (For further details see "WaterWorks", step 1).

Question

Is my heart rate during activity the same on land as it is in water?

Answer

Recent research indicates that heart rates in the water are slightly lower than those reached on land for the equivalent work. While scientific research continues in this area, exercise physiologists suggest that water exercisers can deduct approximately 10 percent from their comparable target heart rate on land.

Question

Can water exercises improve my land sports skills?

Answer

Yes, you can improve your tennis stroke, baseball swing, or soccer kick by practicing these motions in a pool. The water's resistance will help strengthen your swing or kick. The water is an ideal environment to improve any other athletic activity. Don't overlook it. (For a complete program, see my book *The W.E.T. Workout—Water Exercise Techniques*, 1985, New York: Facts on File Publications.)

Question

What kind of bike should I buy? Do I need a ten-speed model in order to receive the benefits of fitness cycling?

Answer

No, you can buy a lightweight, three-speed bike and still reap the cardiovascular benefits from fitness cycling. You can go the same distance on a three-speed as you can on a ten-speed. You don't have to spend a lot of money on a bike; check the newspaper for a secondhand bike.

Question

What are the advantages of using a stationary bicycle?

Answer

Stationary bicycling is an excellent component of your Fitness-Works program. It offers unique advantages. You can exercise at any time, in privacy, regardless of weather conditions. Your risk of injury is small, and because balancing is not your focal point, you can read, listen to music, or watch TV while pedaling. Many serious cyclists use stationary bikes as part of their training program as well as riding their regular bicycles indoors on rollers.

Health, Safety, and BeautyWorks

Question

Can I exercise with a cold?

Answer

You can if the cold is a mild one. You might find that exercise will help you feel better. If you have a fever, you should wait a few days before resuming your exercise program.

Question

When I get sick and I have to stop exercising for a few days, can I start up at the same level once I recover?

Answer

If you miss a few days, you probably can return to your previous level of exercise. If you miss more than four days, it is important that you first get over the illness that is keeping you from exercise. Then resume activity but do about one half or two thirds of what you were doing before you were sick. Let your body be your guide.

Question

At the end of the day, my neck and shoulders feel tight; what can I do to loosen up?

Answer

That tightness is due to a buildup of tension in your neck and shoulders. During your cool-down do head semicircles and shoulder shrugs (described in chapter 2, "StretchWorks").

Question

Why do I feel sore after starting my FitnessWorks program?

Answer

Too much too soon may result in muscle soreness or injury. It is very important to be progressive and consistent, particularly if you are just beginning FitnessWorks. It may take up to eight weeks to build up to a comfortable exercise program. Remember to always warm up and stretch before beginning your main aerobic set. The cool-down helps to remove the waste products (lactic acid) of exercise in the muscle tissue. Listen to your body, and if pain persists, see your doctor.

Question

Sometimes I get a sharp pain in my side when exercising. What is it and what can I do about it?

Answer

A "stitch" can be caused by beginning your main set too quickly and/or breathing improperly. Here, not enough oxygen gets to your muscles and lactic acid, the waste product of exercise, builds up.

Slow your pace down, then inhale and exhale fully. If the stitch is just below your rib cage, stretch your chest and diaphragm muscles by first pressing into the affected area and then raising your arms overhead. When the stitch subsides, continue your workout slowly.

Question

What exercises might cause discomfort or injury?

Answer

Straight leg sit ups, full knee bends, ballistic stretches (bouncing while stretching), and hyperextension (arching) of the back are all possible causes for discomfort or injury.

Injury to muscles and joints can occur as a result of overuse, insufficient warm-up, or jogging on cement or asphalt pavement.

Question

What can I do if I sustain an injury while exercising?

Answer

The best remedy for an exercise-related injury involves *rest, ice, compression,* and *elevation* (or RICE). You need to stop moving and rest the injured area. Apply a cold compress or ice pack wrapped in a towel and wrap it around the muscle with an elastic bandage. RICE helps to keep swelling to a minimum. If the injury is severe, you should see a doctor immediately.

Question

What are the risks of exercising in hot weather?

Answer

In very hot and/or humid weather, there is the risk of heat exhaustion or heat stroke. Heat exhaustion is caused by a depletion of fluids and should be suspected if the body is cold and clammy. Other symptoms include nausea, dizziness, headache, and weak, rapid pulse. Fluids must be replaced immediately. Heat or sun stroke, a more serious condition, occurs when the body's cooling system shuts down. A sign of heat stroke is hot and dry skin. Emergency cooling procedures should be applied immediately: Move the person to a cool place, administer fluids, and call for emergency help. Prevention of overheating depends on drinking plenty of fluids and reducing the amount of exercise during hot weather. Contact your local American Red Cross for instruction on emergency first aid treatment.

Question

How do I protect my skin when exercising?

Answer

You should use an appropriate sunscreen in winter as well as summer months. You should also moisturize your skin both before and after you exercise. Due to perspiration during exercise, women should wear a minimum of makeup when working out.

Question

How can I protect my hair from the elements (wind, sun, water)?

Answer

A bathing cap will help you protect your hair from any chemicals in the water. Remember to shampoo and use a conditioner after each swim. For land FitnessWorks, wear an appropriate hairstyle (with sweatband, sun hat, or clips) to help protect your hair.

Question

Can I exercise during my menstrual period?

Answer

Yes. There are no negative effects to your body when exercising in moderation. In fact, many women who suffer from uncomfortable periods find that exercising can help distract them from cramps or discomfort.

Question

Can I follow the FitnessWorks program during pregnancy?

Answer

Yes, but always check with your physician. If you exercised regularly before your pregnancy and have a normal pregnancy, there should be no problem with continuing to exercise, modifying your workout as your pregnancy progresses. The low-impact FitnessWorks activities of walking, cycling, and swimming are usually recommended for pregnancy.

NutritionWorks

Question

Occasionally I deviate from a low-fat, low-sodium, high-complex carbohydrate diet. Does that mean that I lose all the benefits of the NutritionWorks program?

Answer

If you occasionally eat high-fat or high-sodium foods, you will not lose the benefits of NutritionWorks. However, if you feel your occasional splurge is becoming a regular habit, then corrective measures will be necessary. These splurges may be preventing you from eating the right amounts of the other nutrients you need. You may want to count calories and carefully monitor your intake of carbohydrates, protein, and fat for three typical days to be sure you indeed are following the NutritionWorks program.

Question

What is cellulite and how do I know if I have it?

Answer

Cellulite is another word for body fat. It is uneven distribution of fat deposits. For women, it's usually on the back of the arms and legs where you can't see just how much you have. It's important to be aware of it because in addition to its unsightly appearance, its presence is an indication that you are overweight. To test for it, squeeze the flesh (the outer side of the upper leg is a good spot to check) between thumb and index finger. If the skin looks ripply and lumpy, there is excess fat. Cellulite is reduced by diet and exercise. Unfortunately, even after many people successfully diet, a certain amount of this dimply fat may persist.

Question

What's the best drink to have before and after a workout?

Answer

Water is the best drink to have before, during, if needed, and after your FitnessWorks workout. Your body loses lots of water through perspiration, and the more water you drink during the day, the less likely that you will be dehydrated during a workout. Unlike other liquids, water has the unique quality of being absorbed quickly by your body. You should drink water even if you don't feel thirsty to avoid dehydration.

Some beverages should be avoided before, during, and immediately after a workout. Alcohol constricts the coronary vessels and also acts as a general depressant on the nervous system, thus interfering with coordination, vision, and judgment. Both alcohol and caffeine are diuretics (increase urinary output). Highly sugared beverages can cause stomach and/or intestinal cramping and dehydration during exercise and should also be avoided.

Question
When should I eat before exercising?

Answer
Try eating from one to three hours before exercising to allow your body sufficient time to digest the food. Avoid heavy meals within one hour before your workout.

Question
Why haven't I lost weight since I started exercise?

Answer
You have been building muscle tissue while losing fat. Your body measurements can be reduced even if your weight remains constant because muscle weighs more than fat.

Question
How can I burn more calories during my workout?

Answer
You could increase your speed or intensity of effort, but probably the most effective way is to increase the length of the workout or the total distance. Remember, the number of calories you burn depends on your weight, body composition, activity, and energy efficiency as well as environmental conditions.

Question
Why would two people doing the same activity burn calories at a different rate?

Answer
Besides the fact that each person has a different metabolic rate, people with more muscle tissue burn more calories. In addition, body weight and efficiency (especially in the water) affect your caloric use.

Question
Now that I'm exercising on a regular basis, do I need a vitamin or mineral supplement?

Answer

If you consume a well-balanced diet, your body probably is receiving all the nutrients it needs. However, a multivitamin/mineral supplement that contains approximately 100 percent of the U.S. Recommended Daily Allowance (RDA) can help provide for any inadequacies in your diet. Avoid megavitamins (vitamin and mineral supplements containing many times the RDA). They are usually unnecessary and possibly have toxic effects if taken over long periods of time.

Question

Can women decrease their chances of getting osteoporosis if they consume adequate amounts of calcium?

Answer

Several factors appear to be involved in the prevention of osteoporosis. Research seems to indicate that women who consume large amounts of calcium (approximately 1,000-1,500 mg/day) may decrease their chances of getting osteoporosis. You may want to take calcium supplements if you do not consume enough calcium-rich foods. Research has also indicated that weight-bearing exercise can help prevent the incidence of osteoporosis in females by stimulating the production of new bone tissue. Recently, researchers have cited the decline of estrogen production after menopause as a primary cause of osteoporosis in women.

Question

What foods are high in calcium?

Answer

In addition to milk, cheese, and yogurt, calcium exists in canned salmon with bones, canned sardines with bones, dark green vegetables, and tofu.

Question

How can I control my snack attacks?

Answer

Be aware of how you snack. Nibbles are usually unplanned and uncontrolled, and people often snack while standing in front of an opened refrigerator door. Hundreds of calories can be consumed without your even realizing it. Snacks should be planned ahead, even if only moments before. Eat snacks from a plate, and be sure to sit down and relax while you do so.

Question

I have a variety of health concerns that require me to eat carefully; can I follow the NutritionWorks program?

Answer

The NutritionWorks program was developed for those without any digestive or metabolic disorders. Eat as many Nutrition-Works foods in your diet as your particular condition will allow, and follow the advice of your physician.

Question

Do I have to buy my foods at a health food store to follow the NutritionWorks program?

Answer

No, you don't. Most NutritionWorks foods can be found at your local supermarket. Many supermarkets now carry a line of health foods that is often more reasonably priced than that of health food stores. However, there are foods that you will be able to find mainly in health food stores. Health food stores usually carry a larger selection of the nutritious breads that adhere to NutritionWorks goals as well as a greater variety of whole grain, sugar-free, and salt-free hot and cold cereals.

Question

I'm always in a hurry when I shop. Is there an efficient way to shop in a supermarket?

Answer

Usually, supermarkets are laid out so that fresh food products are on the outside perimeter. Shopping around the edge will help you to avoid most of the processed foods in center aisles and allow you to find meats, produce, and dairy products easily.

Question

Can I use any canned, jarred, or frozen foods?

Answer

Yes, but read the labels carefully before buying them. Remember to avoid sugar, fats, and salt (sodium products). Here are some tips for buying particular canned, jarred, or frozen foods.

Food Item	Best Choice
Tuna fish	Packed in water, unsalted (if it contains salt, rinse thoroughly)
Spaghetti and tomato sauces	No-salt varieties
Jellies, jams, preserves, and conserves	Those prepared without sugar or corn syrup
Frozen vegetables	Plain (no sauce)

Question

Can I ever eat a refined grain product like white bread, cream of wheat, or white rice?

Answer

Yes. They have nutritional value, but be sure to obtain fiber from other foods in your diet.

Question

What should I look for when reading a food label?

Answer

When choosing one product over another, look for the product with the least grams of fat and milligrams of sodium per serving. Ingredients are always listed in descending order of quantity. The first ingredient listed is the predominant ingredient. The last ingredient is the ingredient contained in the least amount. By looking at the ingredients you can get a general idea as to whether the product is overladen with sugar, salt, and oil/fat.

Question

Can I eat pork and lamb, or are they too high in fat?

Answer

In recent years farmers have been producing pork and lamb that is leaner than that of past years. Pork and lamb are red meats and similar in fat content to beef. Trim all visible fat before cooking and blot after cooking. If you eat pork or lamb, include them in your red meat count for the week. (Try not to exceed three servings of red meat per week.)

Question

Are nuts a NutritionWorks food?

Answer

Nuts are a source of protein and minerals, but they are very high in fat. Eat only unsalted varieties. One exception is chestnuts which are very low in fat and can be eaten generously.

Question

Is peanut butter a good food?

Answer

Yes, it contains protein but is high in unsaturated fat. Spread it thin! Choose unsalted, unsweetened peanut butter.

Question

What is the difference between unsaturated and saturated fats?

Answer

In general, vegetable oils (e.g., corn, peanut, safflower, sesame seed, soy bean, olive, and sunflower) are unsaturated (except coconut oil which is saturated) and fats from animals are saturated. At room temperature, saturated fats are solid and polyunsaturated fats are liquid. Both types of fats contain nine calories per gram and should be limited because of this high caloric count. Saturated fat appears to stimulate the body to produce excess cholesterol. Polyunsaturated fats help lower blood cholesterol and therefore are the preferred choice in terms of fat. However, some vegetable oils contain a certain amount of saturated fats (coconut, palm, and cottonseed oil are high in saturated fat). Another type of fat is monounsaturated fat (olive oil and many fish oils contain this type of fat). Some studies have shown that monounsaturated fats are particularly effective in lowering blood cholesterol levels. The general rule, however, is to limit fat intake, but the higher proportion of fat consumed should be poly- or monounsaturated.

Question
Are organ meats good for you?

Answer
Although many organ meats (e.g., kidney, liver, heart) are a good source of protein, vitamins, and minerals, they are high in cholesterol and should be limited.

Question
Can I alter pasta recipes to fit into the NutritionWorks program?

Answer
Yes, very easily. Use whole grain or regular pasta. Alter recipes by

- substituting low-fat and no-salt dairy products,
- limiting oils,
- eliminating sugar and salt, and
- using lean meat.

Question
Are honey and molasses simple sugars?

Answer
Yes, they are; honey and molasses contain trace amounts of vitamins and minerals and should be used, if desired, only in small quantities.

Question
What sweeteners can I use in dessert recipes?

Answer
When choosing dessert recipes, look for recipes using raisins, currants, and dates; date sugar; fruit juices (fresh, canned, or frozen concentrated); fresh fruits (e.g., peaches, pears, apples); sugar-free conserves; and unsweetened canned or frozen fruits. You may find many of the recipes available in books, magazines, and newspapers too sweet. You can experiment by decreasing the amount of sweetener. Aim to use as little sweetener as possible and still get a satisfying taste and texture.

Question
Do I have to eat animal products to get enough protein in my diet?

Answer
Animal products provide us with protein that is complete, meaning it contains the eight essential amino acids. Plant foods, such as grains, beans (lentils), and nuts provide us with incomplete protein. They can provide us with complete protein when eaten in combination with each other. These are called complementary proteins. Some complementary protein combinations are rice and beans, pasta with meat sauce or low-fat cottage cheese, hot or cold cereal with low-fat milk, and peanut butter on whole wheat bread.

Question
Why did starches have such a bad name for so many years?

Answer
There are two reasons. First, little or no distinction was made between simple and complex carbohydrates; people just said carbohydrates are no good for you! Second, starches are often served with condiments containing large amounts of fat such as sour cream, mayonnaise, and butter.

Seek out starches: bread, potatoes, rice, cereals, pasta, beans, peas, popcorn—all foods you thought were fattening and not nutritious. These foods have formed the backbone of great civilizations for thousands of years!

Question

There are foods available that are labeled "cholesterol-free." Does this mean the food is low in fat?

Answer

No, it doesn't. Cholesterol is present only in foods containing animal products. A food can contain a large quantity of vegetable oil and yet be cholesterol-free.

Question

Is margarine a good substitute for butter?

Answer

Although you should limit your use of both, magarine is preferred over butter because it is made from vegetable oils, is more unsaturated, and is cholesterol-free. Also, it spreads more easily than butter, enabling you to use less.

Question

Should children follow the NutritionWorks program?

Answer

Children should not be in the habit of eating fatty, over-salted, and sugary foods. When a child is past the infancy stage, NutritionWorks foods are advisable with the allowance of a somewhat higher percentage of protein and fat. Consult and follow the advice of your pediatrician during your child's growing years.

Question

What do the different sodium labels mean?

Answer

The various labels concerning sodium have the following definitions:

- *Sodium-free* means less than 5 milligrams of sodium per serving.
- *Very low sodium* means 35 milligrams or less of sodium per serving.

- *Low sodium* means 140 milligrams or less of sodium per serving.
- *Reduced sodium* means the food is a substitute for something that contains four times as much sodium.
- *Unsalted, no salt added,* and *without added salt* means the food has been processed without salt and that it is a substitute for a food that is normally processed with salt. Naturally occuring sodium may still be present in some foods.

Question

Should I count calories?

Answer

You may count calories if you are in the habit of doing so, but it is not essential. Just be sure to eat a balanced diet so as to include all the essential nutrients. The important concept is to consume foods that are high in complex carbohydrates, low in sodium, and low in fat. Remember to eat proper servings of each of the four basic food groups. If you follow the NutritionWorks tips your calorie consumption probably will be reduced automatically. Always complement your Nutrition-Works with FitnessWorks.

Question

Do carbohydrates, protein, and fat have the same amount of calories per gram?

Answer

No. Carbohydrates and proteins each have four calories per gram, but fat has nine calories per gram.

Question

How can I find recipes that follow the NutritionWorks program?

Answer

When evaluating recipes you find in magazines and cookbooks, check oil, salt, and sugar ingredient amounts. There are many specialty cookbooks available that offer low-fat, low-sugar, low-sodium, and high-fiber recipes.

Appendix A

SourceWorks

The following organizations are sources to contact for information regarding your different FitnessWorks.

FootWorks

American Hiking Society
1015 31st Street, N.W.
Washington, DC 20007
(703) 385-3252

Education about walking and use of foot trails. Monthly publication.

American Running and Fitness Association
20001 S Street N.W.
Suite 540
Washington, DC 20009
(202) 667-4150

Provides information, motivation, and advice to members and others on running, fitness, and health. Monthly publication.

The Athletics Congress of the U.S.A.
200 South Capitol Avenue
Suite 140
Indianapolis, IN 46225
(317) 638-9155

National governing body for track and field, including Masters events, race walking, and long-distance running. Newsletter available to registered athletes.

New York Road Runners Club
9 East 89th Street
New York, NY 10128
(212) 860-4455

Referral service for competitions, clinics, and medical information. Membership and flyers available.

Walking Association
Box 37228
Tucson, AZ 85740
(602) 742-9589

Works toward the establishment of more walkways and desirable walking standards. Quarterly newsletter available.

Walkways Center
733 15th Street N.W.
Washington, DC 20005
(202) 737-9555

Educates the public about the benefits of walking for fitness, health, and recreation. Publications include annual almanacs and newsletter.

CycleWorks

American Youth Hostels, Inc.
National Administrative Office
P.O. Box 37613
Washington, DC 20013-7613
(202) 783-6161

Sponsors cycling and hiking trips along scenic by-ways. Maintains overnight hostels. Publications include *Hostel Guide* and quarterly magazine. Also, handbooks, travel guides, and accessories available.

Bicycle Federation of America
1818 R Street N.W.
Washington, DC 20009
(202) 332-6986

Promotes increased use of bicycles. Organizes special events. Monthly publication.

BICYCLE USA
League of American Wheelmen
6707 Whitestone Road
Suite 209
Baltimore, MD 21207
(301) 944-3399

Promotes bicycle touring, community education, and club and family cycling. Monthly publication.

Bikecentennial
Box 8308-QG
Missoula, MT 59807
(406) 721-1776

Clearing house for cycling information; develops and maps bicycle routes and promotes recreational cycling. Publications include *Bike Report, Cyclists' Yellow Pages*, and a bimonthly newsletter.

U.S. Cycling Federation
1750 East Boulder Street
Colorado Springs, CO 80909
(303) 578-4581

Governing body of amateur cycling in the United States. Monthly publication.

WaterWorks

American National Red Cross
17th and D Streets N.W.
Washington, DC 20006
(202) 737-8300

Information for aquatics programs and materials. Check your local chapter. Newsletter for aquatic professionals.

Council for National
  Cooperation in Aquatics
901 West New York Street
Indianapolis, IN 46223
(317) 638-4238

Bibliography on all areas of aquatics. Annual meeting and newsletter.

International Swimming Hall
  of Fame
1 Hall of Fame Drive
Fort Lauderdale, FL 33316
(305) 462-6536

Museum of International Aquatics, library, and Olympic aquatic facility available to the public. Provides souvenirs, swim equipment, books, and publications. Clearinghouse for aquatic positions.

National Spa and Pool Institute
2111 Eisenhower Avenue
Alexandria, VA 22314
(703) 838-0083

Establishes standards for design, construction, and operation of pools and spas. Sponsors annual seminars and trade shows for manufacturers. Free materials available to public regarding aquatic safety skills and standards.

U.S. Masters Swimming
National Office
5 Piggott Lane
Avon, CT 06001
(203) 677-9464

Governing body for Masters
and Senior swimming
throughout the United
States. Magazine and newsletter available.

U.S. Swimming, Inc.
1750 Boulder
Colorado Spring, CO 80909
(303) 578-4578

Governing body for amateur
swimming in the U.S.
Monthly publication. In-
cludes *U.S. Swim Newsletter*.

General FitnessWorks

Amateur Athletic Union
3400 West 86th Street
Indianapolis, IN 46268
(317) 872-2900

Governing body for several
amateur sports. Publications
include rulebooks and news-
letters.

American College of Sports
  Medicine
P.O. Box 1440
Indianapolis, IN 46206
(317) 637-9200

Research-related technical information for professionals
concerned with sports
medicine.

American Volkssport
  Association
Suite 203 Phoenix Square
1001 Pat Booker Road
Universal City, TX 78148
(512) 659-2112

Promotes *volkssports*, or noncompetitive, organized
sports, for the health, recreation, and fellowship of the
community. Monthly and bimonthly publication.

Institute for Aerobics Research
12330 Preston Road
Dallas, TX 75230
1-800-527-0362

Researches ways to promote
health through exercise and
diet. Publishes newsletter,
The Aerobic News, which dis-
seminates findings of current
research.

International Association of
  Triathlon Clubs
Cherokee Station
P.O. Box 20427
New York, NY 10028
(212) 288-5661

Seeks to assist and promote
the formation of triathlon
clubs internationally. Bimonthly publication available.

National Fitness Foundation
2250 E. Imperial Highway
Suite 412
El Segundo, CA 90245
(213) 640-0145

Augments existing fitness organizations through educational programs and services for educators, government agencies, corporations, and the general public. Includes the U.S. Fitness Academy.

President's Council on
  Physical Fitness and Sports
Department of Health and
  Human Services
450 5th Street N.W.
Washington, DC 20001
(202) 272-3421

Promotes sports and physical fitness programs. Provides informational materials on exercise and sports for youth, adults, and seniors. Newsletter and program material available.

Sport for Life World
  Headquarters
P.O. Box HM1154
Gibbon Building, Queen Street
Hamilton, Bermuda HMEX
(809) 292-5794

Worldwide organization that provides for all adults to participate in multi-sport festivals, including: World Masters, Games, World Corporate Games, Well-being and Sports Medicine seminars focusing on the mature adult.

United States Jaycees
4 West 21st Street
P.O. Box 7
Tulsa, OK 74121
(918) 584-2481

Provides leadership training for community-based activities through local chapters.

EquipmentWorks

The Finals
21 Minisink Avenue
Port Jervis, NY 12771
1-800-431-9111

Multisport and fitness wear catalogue; mail order available.

Speedo America
The Warnaco Group
7915 Haskell Avenue
Van Nuys, CA 91409
1-800-547-8770

Multisport fitness wear catalog; mail order available.

NutritionWorks

American Cancer Society
4 West 35th Street
New York, NY 10001
(212) 736-3030

Pamphlets available on nutrition and cancer prevention. Check telephone directory for local chapter.

The American Dietetic
  Association
208 South LaSalle
Suite 1100
Chicago, IL 60604-1003
(312) 899-0040

Pamphlets available on general information. Nutrition catalogue listing nutrition books and cookbooks also available. Check telephone directory for local association. Referrals to agencies and dieticians available through local offices.

The American Heart
  Association
National Center
7320 Greenville Avenue
Dallas, TX 75231
(214) 750-5300

Materials available on nutrition and exercise to promote health. Check telephone directory for local chapter.

Department of Health and
  Human Services
Human Nutrition Information
  Services
United States Department of
  Agriculture
6505 Belcrest Road
Room 325 A
Federal Building
Hyattsville, MD 20782
(301) 436-8617

Nutritional materials available. A list of publications is available and can be ordered direct. Some publications are free and for some there is a nominal charge.

Food and Nutrition
  Information Center
National Agricultural Library
10301 Baltimore Boulevard
Room 304
Beltsville, MD 20705
(301) 344-3719

Publishes *Pathfinders*: listings of short bibliographies of books about nutrition and sports medicine. Books are categorized by levels: consumer, educational, and professional. Books can be borrowed at public libraries via interlibrary loan.

U.S. Department of Health and
Human Services
Food and Drug Administration
5600 Fishers Lane-HFE88
Rockville, MD 20852
(301) 443-3170

Nutritional materials available upon request; these materials can be reproduced. Information can be requested by postcard for specific topic. Available publications will be sent to you.

Appendix B

FitnessWorks™ Training Log

FitnessWorks Training Log

Date	Resting Pulse	FitnessWorks Activity	Warm-Up Pulse	Main Set Pulse	Cool-Down Pulse	Total Time/ Distance	Comments

Index